A Novel Approach to Healing

by

Angela cng Delglyn

Dedication

This book is dedicated to all the friends and clients who've stimulated, changed or added to my thinking, and ultimately encouraged yet more thinking and investigation.

Publisher Links:

http://www.satinpaperbacks.com

http://www.satinpublishing.co.uk

https://twitter.com/SatinPaperbacks

https://www.facebook.com/Satinpaperbackscom

Email: nicky.fitzmaurice@satinpaperbacks.com

Author links:

https://www.facebook.com/In-Form-Optimal-Health-110719832291329/?ref=hl

Visit: www.in-form.co.uk

In Form Optimal Health is the website through which Angela offers specialised massage, Channelled Coaching and Soul Plan readings.

What others are saying about 'A Novel Approach to Healing'

"An insightful read, following the long and sometimes lonely journey of a 'sensitive', which eventually leads to her ultimate realisation and understanding of 'WHY?'" Corinna L-K

"I found the bio of great interest, but then the story gave way to deeper meanderings that left me wondering where I was in my own life. That may have been a reflection of my deeper self, because on subsequent readings, I have been able to see aspects of myself show themselves where previously I may not have been willing to accept them. If this was indeed the purpose of this book, then it has been successful in gently pointing these things out for me explore further when I am ready. As for the A-Z, I found that a useful array of health-related topics that I can dip into as and when I need to. Many of the symptoms listed resonated and left me thinking about the treatments she suggests. This book has left me musing about life in general, and me, my body, mind and spirit in particular." TM

"There is a great moral tale within Angela's book, and that is when life becomes hard to handle, don't wait for the situation to deteriorate to a level where you are left exhausted and unable to cope. It's also about self-help and recognising the problems you are storing up both physically and mentally.

This is not just a book of a woman's quest for answers, it is a book for those determined to change the course of their life because they are willing to move forward by trying something different and new." Michael C.

Intellectual Acknowledgement:

By www.seqlegal.com

Introduction

We will not be liable to you in respect of any losses arising out of any event or events beyond our reasonable control. This disclaimer governs the use of this Book. By using this Book, you accept this disclaimer in full.

Credit

This disclaimer was created using an SEQ Legal template.

No advice

The Book contains information about health care. The information is not advice, and should not be treated as such.

You must not rely on the information in this Book as an alternative to medical advice from an appropriately qualified professional. If you have any specific questions about any medical matter you should consult an appropriately qualified professional.

If you think you may be suffering from any medical condition you should seek immediate medical attention. You should never delay seeking medical advice, disregard medical advice, or discontinue medical treatment because of information in the Book.

You should never delay seeking legal advice, disregard legal advice, or commence or discontinue any legal action because of information in the Book.

No representations or warranties

To the maximum extent permitted by applicable law and

subject to section 6 below, we exclude all representations, warranties, undertakings and guarantees relating to the Book.

Without prejudice to the generality of the foregoing paragraph, we do not represent, warrant, undertake or guarantee:

- that the information in the Book is correct, accurate, complete or non-misleading;
- that the use of the guidance in the Book will lead to any particular outcome or result; or
- in particular, that by using the guidance in the Book you will realise greater health benefits.

Limitations and exclusions of liability
The limitations and exclusions of liability set out in this section and elsewhere in this disclaimer are subject to section 6 below and govern all liabilities arising under the disclaimer or in relation to the Book, including liabilities arising in contract, in tort (including negligence) and for breach of statutory duty.

We will not be liable to you in respect of any business losses, including without limitation loss of or damage to profits, income, revenue, use, production, anticipated savings, business, contracts, commercial opportunities or goodwill.

We will not be liable to you in respect of any special, indirect or consequential loss or damage.

Exceptions
Nothing in this disclaimer shall: limit or exclude our liability for death or personal injury resulting from negligence; limit

or exclude our liability for fraud or fraudulent misrepresentation; limit any of our liabilities in any way that is not permitted under applicable law; or exclude any of our liabilities that may not be excluded under applicable law.

Severability

If a section of this disclaimer is determined by any court or other competent authority to be unlawful and/or unenforceable, the other sections of this disclaimer continue in effect.

If any unlawful and/or unenforceable section would be lawful or enforceable if part of it were deleted, that part will be deemed to be deleted, and the rest of the section will continue in effect.

Law and jurisdiction

This disclaimer will be governed by and construed in accordance with English law, and any disputes relating to this disclaimer will be subject to the exclusive jurisdiction of the courts of England and Wales.

Our details

In this disclaimer, "we" means (and "us" and "our" refer to) Angela Delglyn trading as In Form – Optimal Health, who can be contacted via www.in-form.co.uk.

Acknowledgements

First, I'd like to acknowledge my boys - Ryan and Mark - through whom I've learned so much since the day they were born.

To the memory of my friend and mentor, David Perry, for his guidance and kind encouragement in the early years, not to mention introducing me to dowsing.

To Dawn Golten for her help, support and friendship whilst getting my business up and running in the south.

To Sheri Dixon for her teaching, patience and friendship. Looking back, I realise that my time of study with Sheri was a significant turning point and I value her input tremendously, both at and since that time.

To my dear friend Susannah Todd for helping me discover the finer points of formatting and layout.

To my good friends - Marilyn, Corinna, Claudia, Samira and Frank for their unfailing friendship and belief in me during this project.

These people have all inadvertently contributed to drawing out the many random facts and bits of wisdom that I possess in order that they be seen for what they are - a series of sign posts that others can follow if they so desire

Table of Contents

Preface

The dilemma that today's humans face is how to live in a material world, full of man-made detritus, whilst having access to the most amazing gifts that nature has to offer. Over time, the disconnection between these two worlds increases; we are given the choice to pick the fruits of either, and yet all too often we fail to flourish. There is immense confusion about what actually nourishes us in this modern world. Many people are rendered powerless by this confusion, and as a result exist on a muddled autopilot for a good deal of the time, while they feel their potential quietly slipping away.

Deep within each and every one of us are the foundational tools that provide us with the skills necessary to navigate this world, and all it may offer. This is the story of how one person explored those tools and natural skills and began the continual process of honing her instinct to a fine point whilst defining her own healing path. That process of questioning and defining became all-important in order to create a strong foundation of repeatable processes that would serve to navigate the obstacles of the modern world, and in that way achieve health and wellbeing whilst living in it. What became apparent is that this process is never complete – it cannot be – for as change continues to happen, so too must the strategy to adapt and adopt new ways of being and doing, in every aspect of life.

Being curious, looking beyond the words of others and delving deeply into what each experience offered brought forward a personal truth that now paves the way to the limitless potential supported by that foundation.

PART I

In the beginning...

A dim and distant memory hung with some significance over the first 35 years of my life. This memory presented in the form of a repetitive dream where I was playing happy and content within a cosy confined space that I later came to realise was the womb. Eventually, my contentment was disturbed by the prompt - "It's time" - time to leave that cosy, warm, protected place and enter the wider world.

With a very heavy heart, as if sensing the tone of what was to come, I knelt down and placed the top of my head into the confined exit...

1

Setting the scene

The memories of my early years are a catalogue of sensations – what I experienced by way of my senses – all the events that began to shape me since my first breath. Obviously, some are more memorable than others and so stand out, but the trail of sensations was real enough and all helped to form who I became.

I was born into a large farming family in rural North Staffordshire – not that remote, but far enough away from the village to keep us from pursuing a natural curiosity away from home. Living on a farm meant there was always something of interest to experience or investigate, and if that wasn't enough, there were plenty of siblings to play with or dodge.

In those days, we weren't kept cooped up in the house very much, but were prone to wandering like free-range hens, thus encountering odd moments of disaster. For instance, around the age of 3 or 4, it seemed like a 'Right of Passage' to fall into a cattle drinking trough or a pond, only to be plucked out in the nick of time, none the worse for wear. Strangely none of us remember those times.

Once I was sitting swinging on a bit of chicken wire fence when I fell backwards, banging my head hard on the stone churn stand, cutting it open an inch or so.

One of the workmen came running and scooped me up – he'd heard the bump from a way off and took me into the house where the blood and tears were dabbed away; nothing to worry about then, eh?

Another time, my sister, wearing steel toe-capped boots, kicked me so hard on the shin that my leg broke. She must have made a speedy exit as she doesn't remember it now, but I do – I was inconsolable for hours. I can't remember much about lugging around a full-leg plaster cast at the age of 3, I guess I mostly sat. However, the break caused a deep ache in that leg for many years when I went to bed, worse when the weather was changing, and I'd often cry myself to sleep with the pain. I was relieved when the leg had grown enough to improve the circulation and the ache went away.

Sometime around the age of 12, I recall having a kidney infection. The pain was immense; I couldn't move my torso in any way without excruciating pain. This lasted for about a week, but there was no doctors' visit. Whatever happened in the kidney at that time left its mark as I seemed to suffer problems in my left kidney for several decades during the turn of the seasons.

I recall how we had a rope swing rigged up in one of the hay sheds, whereby the challenge was to see how high you could get while swinging on it.

Unfortunately, during one of these escapades, my competitive nature meant that I crashed backwards into one of the brick pillars, hitting my head very hard. I suffered headaches and neck problems for many a while after that, and whilst using a foam pillow in bed helped to some degree, the problem persisted for many years. Greater relief was only found years later as I began to investigate osteopathic and chiropractic treatments and some of the damage was unravelled.

The inevitable contagion of diseases like measles, mumps and chicken pox were of course present, but other incidentals like low blood sugar, repeated earache and tonsillitis added to the physical burden.

Looking back

The list of physical challenges above that I experienced whilst growing up are not totally exhaustive, but whatever the cause, all of these problems laid a foundation for who I grew into, on the physical, mental and emotional levels, setting the tone for the new challenges I was to meet in adulthood.

According to the writings of Dr Bruce Lipton (The Honeymoon Effect), up to the age of seven years, we automatically 'download' from our family and immediate surroundings the experiences upon which we form our core belief systems. These belief systems become the main program that we run from our subconscious mind until such a time as we see fit to consciously change it. As most people generally only work from their conscious mind for about 15% of the day, the rest of the time is spent running on the original program. Our original program may be full of misperceptions and misinformation thus making the foundation from which we act/react somewhat flawed, but that can be hard to see from the inside. The reason Dr Lipton called his book The Honeymoon Effect is because he states that we can make our thinking more conscious - like when we are falling in love – and thus develop a new program for a new way of being. Much of the current mindfulness movement has sprung from this idea.

Phase One 16 – 33 yrs

After leaving the routine of school life, I had really wanted to go on to art school, but at the time didn't feel I could because I was conditioned to believe that money was always an issue. So with a lack of discussion about my future, I decided to ask a friends' father for a job at the nearby Building Society in order to begin earning. As he already knew my family, the interview was a formality, and I entered the corporate world on the first rung of the ladder.

From those fumbling early days of work, where I became acquainted with more people than I'd ever known before, my life became much more interesting, more colourful, and well, just *more*. My expanded world suddenly contained many more choices and possibilities of what to do with my time. Of course, it took me a while to learn how to handle my newfound money, not having been taught or used to that sort of thing, but I was usually able to find enough outlets for my energy and sense of fun that my budget could stretch to, including my beloved dancing.

At the tender age of 19, I married and found myself toting a mortgage for the first time in my life. On paper, this wasn't so bad, after all there were two of us, and we were both working. What I hadn't bargained for was that my newly wedded husband was bi-polar, and how that would place a massive strain upon our marriage. From the off, there were frequent repair bills for the cars he'd crashed during his mania, not to mention the numerous fines. Then there were the 'impulse buys' that ran up huge debts and his nightly visits to the pub, even when he was out of a job. At one point, I found myself, as the main breadwinner, in the position of deciding whether to buy a loaf of bread or a pint of milk with the money in my purse. Thank goodness for the resilience of youth!

Now, it puzzles me as I look back upon that first decade of my marriage, how it was that I failed to realise the importance of eating wholesome, live, nourishing foods, despite having been reared on home grown food from our farm. I can only assume that when we enter the wider world and begin our ascent up the ladder of life, that there are just too many new experiences to process and consider, and that as long as hunger is satisfied in that moment, then everything is okay. I know that at the time, I certainly didn't understand the mechanics of food and was therefore lacking in my ability to take good care of myself. However, I survived, as many of us do in these situations, but I would not say that I thrived.

The marriage dragged on for 13 long years, during which time I steadily ascended the career ladder at work, *and* managed to add other fields of interest to my existing knowledge. However, the toll of trying to build a fulfilling life with a bi-polar husband *and* do shift work for many years became too much, and my energy levels took a determined down turn.

At first, I propped myself up on ginseng, but the feeling of my eyes being 'out on sticks' was not for me. Eventually a work colleague told me about an eminent herbalist not too far away, and so I went to see her. It seemed the consequences of all that I'd been through, put up with and worked at had exhausted my adrenals, and that many of the normal functions of my body had become weak. I had become consciously acquainted with the mark of stress.

The herbalist taught me Autogenics, which helped initially to reduce the stress levels. However, my energy was still very low. In the final 2 years of my marriage, I would go to work, manage a few 'normal' hours of work, and then rush home at lunchtime for a microwave meal and a 20-minute power nap on the floor. If for some reason I couldn't get home at lunchtime, I would have to find an empty meeting room where I could lie down on the floor for 10 minutes just so that I could get through the afternoon. I felt permanently exhausted during that unhappy time, with very little to uplift or fulfil me – although some revelry with a girl friend at work provided a welcome distraction. Eventually, I realised I couldn't go on like that and began to consider a career change.

The seed of change took a year to germinate before I made the decision to study remedial massage. I had to fund the course myself, which meant an agonising year of remaining in a job I no longer wanted to do, and a marriage I no longer wanted to be a part of. As someone who likes to act quickly upon her decisions, I found that year very hard, so I was grateful for the support of a good friend who kept me focused on my goal.

During my course, I was staying at a Bed and Breakfast for my first practical study weekend, when I had what I can only describe as a brainstorm; I made the decision, with a great sense of clarity, to end my marriage. Unfortunately, the housing market was in a major crisis and our house took 2 years to sell, finally making only a quarter of it's former worth, so there was to be no speedy exit. Maybe it was the strain of living in the same house as someone I no longer had any faith in, or maybe it was my brains way of saying "enough!" but during that year I began to suffer black-outs where I'd be 'unconscious' for 12-18 hours at a time. Anxiety attacks interspersed the blackouts until finally concrete change occurred.

I left my IT job as soon as I became a qualified therapist, and set about building a practice in a draughty room above a gymnasium in my local town. Although massage is now quite commonplace and well received, it certainly wasn't the case in those days. My practice was the first of its kind in a hard-bitten town, so I had a few curious fellows popping their heads round the door to question what I was offering ... needless to say, they were given short shrift! However, on the up side, I had an amazing year where I saw a great variety of different conditions from which to learn. I confess to having a rather useful asset to aid my learning though – I would often acquire the pain of the client who was coming to see me 3 days before they arrived, so always 'just knew' exactly where to treat and how, to the puzzlement of many.

So as one phase of my life concluded, the scene was effectively set for the next that was to last almost as long.

What had I learned so far?
Whilst still in my teens, the mechanics of the body had already begun to interest me. I watched a very lithe lady in a pale blue leotard doing yoga on TV and so experimented with it myself – something I still continue with today in order to satisfy my innate need to stretch.

Around the time I was wed at the tender age of 19, there was a downturn in my diet and, coupled with a hormonal imbalance triggered by the contraceptive pill, I gained a lot of weight between my waist and knees. One day, I caught a glimpse of my permanent knicker line, visible through ever-tightening jeans, being reflected back to me from a shop window, and I realised how my shape had changed. So I bought an Elancyl massager, complete with ivy extract bar(!) and set to work on smoothing out my thighs. While it did help, balancing the hormones was ultimately more effective, but that was yet to come.

A couple of decades later, after studying Deep Lymphatic Therapy, my thoughts returned to the 'Elancyl principle' whilst investigating ways to stimulate the lymphatic system. I considered the structure of the lymphatics in the broken leg I'd sustained at three years of age, and how the effect of the damage would never completely go away. My training had enlightened me as to how lymph can build up and solidify in certain circumstances, but I also wondered if this generally occurred around fatty deposits in weight gain too. This and other questions would in later years contribute to me working out an easy system of self-help for stimulating the lymphatic system of anyone who would care to try.

Aside from these physical insights, I had learned that despite my inner strength, I was not immune to the ravages of stress, and how it had depleted my body more than I could envisage at the time. I had had first-hand experience of living in a way that did not nourish me – either mentally, physically or emotionally. I learned that stress is a major obstacle that inhibits good health; I had also learned that the huge amounts of energy required to live that kind of life can not be sustained.   More importantly, I'd endured many personal experiments on how to 'be'... or not.

Phase Two 33 – 54 yrs

The second phase of my life began with great alacrity in the form of a new relationship and, soon after, my first pregnancy. Sadly, that first failed at 6 weeks, but a few months later, my second pregnancy seeded successfully. Interestingly, just prior to the pregnancy, I had endured an 18-month period of being vegan under the guidance of the afore-mentioned herbalist. Although the purpose of the vegan diet was to heal a leaky gut, that style of eating really didn't suit me – I was always cold, hungry and constipated and lacking energy so I was glad to revert to my naturally omnivorous state.

In order to better accommodate the new arrival in our lives, we moved from a town flat to a sweet little country cottage on the edge of Shropshire, complete with roses around the front door. I was about 6 months pregnant when we moved there so still had time to enjoy working on the garden and exploring the walks in the area with our Doberman dog. By this time, I was being much more careful about my diet and was supplementing with Superfood or spirulina stirred into yoghurt - a taste I endured, rather than acquired. Some years later, I was amused to notice that my son actually liked the grim taste of the spirulina I'd consumed whilst I carried him.

At the time my son was born, he was found to have the umbilical cord around his neck, so his head and upper body were blue, and a spell in the incubator was necessary. I was told there was no apparent harm done, but it transpired that he didn't sleep for more than 2 hours at a time for the next 2 years and seemed too afraid to be left alone. This was quite a strain on me and I naturally became exhausted. Unwittingly I conceived again, and our second son was born 17 months after the first. At the time of his birth, I was too tired to keep food down and could barely manage to hold him. It came as no surprise then that I couldn't supply sufficient breast milk and had to resort to formula instead.

When our first son was 6 months old, his father decided to set up his own business. This meant he was frequently away from home so, apart from time at weekends, I was effectively a single mother and our baby felt he'd lost the parent he had bonded with. During that time we had one car which was used for work purposes, so I had to manage with the local bus service into town for shopping whilst juggling the baby, buggy and all the bags.

When our second son came along, my energy was seriously flagging, so we decided to move back to the locality of my family, in order for me to have some support. I managed to procure a heavy second-hand twin chariot for the babes to ride in, so I could push them up the hill and into town for their early social life. Upon our return at lunchtime, I'd feed the three of us then stagger up the stairs with a child tucked under each arm for a desperately needed nap. My mind doggedly kept me putting one foot in front of the other, doing what was needed on a daily basis, but all the while wearing the harness of perpetual tiredness.

Sometime later, while the boys were still quite small, my partner bought our first house in a nearby village, and for a while we were happy there as we nested and made home, and our eldest began school. However, as time moved on and the tiredness was still present, it was evident that something was wrong. It was early 1996, and I had embarked upon another course of study. I was trying to complete a question paper and would find that the sentences I was constructing in my mind would keep vanishing, my concentration was non-existent; I could no longer think.

My older sister gave me a seminar booklet about Myalgic Encephalomyelitis, convinced that this was my problem. I read the booklet and agreed it sounded plausible, but nevertheless, took it to my doctor for her comments. Sadly, she confessed to knowing nothing about the subject and dismissed me with the advice to follow my own beliefs. I was very disheartened, as I really wanted support, and there wasn't much information around at the time, the Internet not being what it is today. This condition lasted for about two and a half years until circumstances called for action. However later that year, we moved house again, this time to a much bigger place, and I did what my sparse energy allowed to help make the place ours. The boys loved all the space that we had; it was indeed a lovely home.

1998 was a difficult year. Sadly, my partner, for whatever reasons only he could fathom, had become paranoid and convinced that I was 'up to no good' whilst he was out at work, despite me suffering from chronic fatigue. He took to spying on me with various devices (some of which I found and smashed) and making wild accusations that systematically trashed my reputation throughout friends and family. Had I not had two lovely boys to care for, I doubt whether I'd still be here.

The physical abuse began a short while later, so I grabbed the boys and made a speedy get away using a spare set of car keys I'd hidden in the front garden, having no choice but to return to my family. Of course, that was a big shock to my partner, and Peggs flower shop had a bumper week, but it wasn't practical to stay with the family for long and so we went back. When it happened again, I knew I had to get out, but I didn't know how to go about it. Strangely, events unfolded before me and an opportunity came up that was actually presented by 'Himself'; he called it a 'window of opportunity' through which I could escape. I grabbed the chance with both hands, valuing my safety above all else, and in the process, like a rabbit caught in headlights, I signed away all rights to any equity in the property that I had helped create, although I was *allowed* to keep the furniture and my car.

So I was on the move again, not far this time, just up the road to borrow the house that my brother was getting ready for him and his girlfriend, but at least free of the tyrant my partner had become. Whilst it was a sad situation, one of the good things about having children is that they make you dig ever deeper within yourself to pull out reserves you never knew you had, and for that I am grateful. We stayed there for about six months, until my brother needed his house back and we had managed to procure a place closer to the boys' school. We could only get a 6-month tenancy there so we had to move *again* to a house across the street, where we stayed for two happy years, during which time I regained some of my lost energy and confidence. Somewhere around this time, I noticed the first signs of hormonal imbalance in the guise of hot flushes, something that would continue in varying degrees for well over a decade.

Late in 1998, a surprising feeling of *needing* to move developed within my solar plexus - surprising because moving is exhausting, so why on earth would I want to do it again if it wasn't necessary? This feeling was new and different to me, but it grew in intensity until one day, as I sat in the spiritualist church that my uncle and aunt ran, the medium pointed at me from the podium and shouted;

"You – what are you still doing here? You should be in the South!"

Interestingly, this comment corroborated what I'd felt but was unable to gain any clarity on, so I agreed with him before returning to my mild frustration of not knowing how to respond to my gut feeling. Of course, more waiting was the answer, because events did indeed create the opening I'd been seeking, and in January 2001 I made the move to leafy Hertfordshire – alone.

The relationship that was my 'stepping-stone' sank within a few months of the move, so having nowhere else to live; I had a few weeks of living-in at the place where I worked. Simultaneously, my boys' father decided to vanish, apparently feeling that he couldn't cope with the emotional demands of his children and being their main carer. This meant that my weekend trips back to the north took on a new emphasis. A family pow-wow ensued with plenty of mutterings as my tribe tried to apply the necessary pressure to bring me back. However, I saw things somewhat differently and thought more in terms of moving the boys to be with me. I'd worked hard to get a new practice up and running within a month of being in Hertfordshire and I wasn't about to give that up. It had become apparent to me that there were far more opportunities in the south than where we came from, and I believed with a bit of effort, I could make anything happen, and I did.

The earnings from my new business, and the money I got from a part-time job meant that I could make a decent home for my boys whilst establishing them in their new routines. My youngest took a long time to settle, and we had several bouts of head lice from school (according to Louise Hay, parasites are about giving away one's power to others, letting them take over), something we'd not experienced previously. Nevertheless we delighted in building our new life together as a team.

It wasn't long before the boys found some playmates on the close, including one slightly older boy who was visiting his father. My two invited him into our house and they became lost in a world of play until his father tracked him to my door. An interesting way to meet someone, and not one I'd envisaged, but the father and I soon began to see more of each other. Nine months later, I moved in with him, partly for practical reasons, but also because it 'seemed' like the right thing to do at the time. It was strange then that I couldn't make sense of the tears that flowed all day as we moved into his house - was my subconscious was trying to tell me something?

The boys settled happily into their new home, glad to be under the auspices of this big, affable man, and I too seemed relaxed. We were getting along well and nothing too horrendous cropped up in over a year, so we decided to be wed; just a small affair with a handful of our friends. Sometime later, there was an argument over a speeding ticket that my husband acquired whilst driving my car. He had me take the rap for it and I later found he'd done this with a previous wife; I was astounded and angry that I had been put in such a position. Maybe that was the beginning of our demise, but a change certainly set in after that, and we fell to bickering. The bickering continued and try as I might to work out what and why, I failed to improve things. The situation became untenable for me, and I knew that if I was to stay emotionally intact, I had to leave.

It was relatively easy to manifest a house to rent in the next town, but less so to move the boys to a new school. My first application for a place was refused, but with determination I managed to successfully navigate the appeals process. For the first year, I was to and fro between schools, having one boy in each town, until the crinkles of that stressor eased out.

Again, all seemed well and my team were happy once more. Unfortunately, our next-door neighbours seemed bent on changing that with late night bonfires that sent smoke in through our windows and making noise aplenty whilst we were trying to sleep, not to mention nosey, which is relevant when you're a highly sensitive and private being like me.

Exasperated, we moved again, but this time to a delightful little cottage near the canal. We had country walks from the doorstep and a garden to die for, and enjoyed six happy years there.

Sadly though, within a year of moving in, my health began to deteriorate and problems with my digestive system and hormones prevailed. My small intestine would become very sore and distended for several days at a time, and my energy was elusive, eventually worsening to the point where I was unable to work. I was saddened and frustrated that my visits to the doctor were met with derision instead of help, so again I set about doing research of my own to look for answers.

The 'whys' didn't come easily (I found myself wondering what someone with zero nutritional knowledge would do) but I persisted. Firstly, I discovered through the writings of Walter Last that the main reason for my intestinal distension was due to fat mal-absorption. I am uncertain as to the precise reason for having this condition, although my guess would be a genetic element. I recall hearing of other relatives having similar problems too and when coupled with the effect of the high-fibre diet I'd been used to and its irritation to the gut wall, I was starting to make sense of the situation. The effect was bulky, odorous stools, which over time had led me to be deficient in several essential fatty acids, vitamins and minerals.

Indeed, it was not long after this realization that I noticed the skin of my neck, belly, inner thighs and backs of my arms sagging like a 90 year old, yet I wasn't even 50! At the time this was a big shock and I had no idea what to do, but one day I was playing an audiotape that a friend had lent to me and I heard the speaker talking about the *visual* signs of magnesium deficiency. He clearly described the saggy skin, something I'd not previously read in any textbook or research materials. Of course, this information enabled me to correct the problem relatively quickly and my skin resumed its normal elasticity.

So, armed with the result of my research and the seeking of direction through my contacts, I tracked down a wonderful lady with a wealth of knowledge whom I now consider to be significant in helping to turn my life around. I was so impressed by the diversity of her knowledge and advice that I decided to train with her and became certified as a metabolic typing (MT) advisor. Time studying the subject material was only the beginning; drip-fed wisdom arrived over the ensuing years as a result of the understanding and my further experimentation that I had pursued. Looking back, I began to understand more about the impact of the prolonged stress upon my body and how the systems and functions had been weakened from the duress.

After discussions with my teacher, I also took the decision to go onto HRT patches; my hormonal imbalances had become so bad that at times I struggled to climb the stairs let alone work, and the natural means of support I'd been trying were pathetically lacking. It was simply ridiculous to think that I could carry on as I had been. It turned out that I only needed the HRT for 5 years before my body let me know that it was enough, and I've since managed to balance my hormones with sporadic use of pregnenolone, evening primrose oil and a small amount of progesterone, dowsing my needs around my normal cycle. I continue to use this protocol today, along with Maca (a ground Peruvian root with adaptogenic qualities) but seem to need it less as time goes by, as long as I keep stress to a minimum.

During this time, I spent a good deal of time studying liver function and I came to understand the importance of the role it plays in bringing balance to the body. It is fair to say that when any system of the body is out of kilter, the liver carries an extra load, as well as its normal work, whilst trying to support a return to normal function. I had suffered many symptoms of a burgeoning liver on and off for some time from the distended abdomen, sluggish digestion, intolerance to alcohol and rich foods, sore gritty eyes, broken sleep, greasy itchy scalp to name a few. For quite a while, I thought the answer to all my problems must therefore lie in *how* my liver was functioning. It was another few years before I realised that my liver function was fine, it was just doing the work of three livers, so I dug down even deeper until I later found what I now believe to be the real answer to my health problems.

During the ensuing years, I continued to experiment with the effects of different foods, their combinations and a few key supplements based upon the teaching I'd received and my own research. I observed my energy levels, moods, emotions and overall wellbeing, getting to really know their range. One of the biggest surprises in those early days of experimentation was how eating something starchy (without protein) made me sleepy within 20 minutes! I have since put this information to good use by avoiding grain starches at lunch time when I need to be productive so that I can continue to stay alert during the afternoon.

Over time, I was to understand a lot more about how to support and balance my system, not just throughout the day, but the over the weeks and months, as a way of continually maintaining good health, not just through food, but by knitting together all facets of living.

These happy years saw my boys finish school, start jobs and begin to develop and expand their own lives upon their chosen pathways. It was indeed a wonderful platform for growth and change in all our lives and the many happy memories from those days will remain in each of our hearts for many years.

What did I learn at this time?

One of the best changes I made upon embarking on my MT training was to supplement betaine HCl – stomach acid. Within a few days of starting, my gut began to settle down and no longer produced the gas that had created so much discomfort over the years (frequently ascribed as an IBS symptom by many people). I learned that the lack of acidity in my stomach meant it did not support proper digestion throughout the GI tract, and I was therefore not breaking down my food effectively (hence the fermentation/gas production), *or* assimilating it efficiently (hence the lack of energy). On top of that, my internal condition had created an environment *where candida could thrive* – none of which had anything to do with the quality of my diet.

25

Another helpful factor that I learned during this time was how the husks of grains and seeds can irritate the gut of a para-sympathetic dominant, as I was (the sympathetic and para-sympathetic nervous systems are branches of the Autonomic Nervous System - see the Balancing Act chapter for more information). As I'd been in the habit for some years of enjoying the reported 'wholesomeness' of whole wheat bread and seeds of all kinds, including psyllium, this was a significant discovery. As soon as I removed the whole grains and seeds from my diet, my gut was able to heal. Once whilst abroad, a friend made me lunch before I made the journey home and offered me some flatbread that she'd made in her dehydrator; the problem was it was full of seeds. I hesitated as I held the piece of flatbread and my gut gave a spasm which I later realised was my body's signal of how it would respond if I ate it. Well, I ate the flatbread out of politeness and regretted it for the whole journey home, with stomach cramps aplenty. Lesson learned.

The third important factor I learned at this time was how to regulate my fluctuating blood sugar levels. I realised after using a glucometer for a while, that I didn't even recognise what stable blood sugar felt like! (These days, I notice how many people's hands tremble with low blood sugar, and I don't mean old people!) My teacher helped me to understand that only by balancing every meal *and* snack could I achieve the stability I'd been missing. Now, after years of eating consciously, I no longer have to question my blood sugar level, I *know* how it feels, and my body tells me if it's not had what it needs to feel good.

Phase Three 54-56yrs

As the boys geared up to go solo, I knew that changes were on the way for me too, and once again I got the calling from spirit to get ready for another big move. For quite some time I had no idea where it was going to be, but eventually I was 'shown' somewhere I'd been to before and therefore recognised the beautiful city of Bath. I was impressed, despite not having the faintest idea of the agenda.

A massive sifting of my possessions took place, and I jettisoned anything that I didn't think I'd need again, as I'd already 'seen' the 3rd floor flat that I would be occupying. I also made sure that I tied up all loose ends to my past; I wanted to be totally free of limitation, and ready for whatever dramatic change was on the cards. As the details of the planned move fell into place, my anticipation and excitement grew as I envisaged this new phase of my life.

Around this time, a handsome young man I'd met briefly at a local dance asked me out. We met just a couple of times before the eve of the move arrived. I recall packing late into that evening before rushing out to catch the last hour at the local venue and what I thought would be my last dance with him. Despite the fact that we barely knew each other, his attempts to hide his feelings were only partially successful and I was surprised to sense his anger at my leaving. Still, I didn't have time to dwell on that, I had a grand move to take care of, so we said our goodbyes and went our separate ways.

The next day, the early arrival of the removal men meant I had more than enough to think about, and it wasn't until they'd left and I was checking around that I realised I'd forgotten to defrost the freezer. After what seemed an interminable delay, I dropped off the keys to our happy home and hit the road, driving the 2-hour journey down to my sisters' place for the night.

The following morning, I was up and out early, knocking on the estate agents' door in Bath at 9am, ready to finalise paperwork and collect the keys. A snooty young man, wearing the traditional Agents' garb of tight-fitting shiny suit and pointy shoes, was the only person in the office and the transition was somewhat less than smooth. However, I ran back down the road with a light heart, ready to enter my new life in Bath with gusto.

Downsizing from a 3 bed cottage into a 2 bed flat requires a stringent use of space, so I was truly dismayed to find the kitchen cupboards still full of the last tenants pots and pans, and not even clean at that. As fast as I tried to think of what to do, the space around me was rapidly being filled with boxes, as the removal men efficiently proved their worth. My sister came to the rescue with a plan and between us we transferred the unwanted things into the boxes we had just emptied whilst somehow cleaning and putting away my stuff, rather like one of those plastic puzzles where you shuffle the squares around to make the picture. In a room the width of a corridor, and with floor space disappearing fast, this was not as simple as it sounded.

Somehow we got through the worst of the day, until I'd just had enough and was on the verge of tears, so I asked everyone to leave. It transpired the removal chaps were hanging around en-masse expecting a large tip, but all I could see were too many people at a time when I was feeling completely overwhelmed. The effort of this move had been considerably more than any other I'd done. I realised that every move I'd ever made had required me to dig ever deeper inside myself, drawing upon and using some of my personal power to make it happen. Whilst I still had my boys as a reason to strive, I could do it, but when it was just for me, it seemed so much harder. The process was exhausting – mentally, physically and emotionally – and I needed time for my internal well to refill.

⌘

The bright light of the mid-summer mornings streaming in through the tall Georgian windows, played its part in refilling my well a little more each day as I made home in Bath. One day I sat in my armchair looking out across the valley and had a flashback to a dream I'd had at least 2 years previously; I had 'seen' this view before and had even tried to paint it. There were other similar instances where my presence in Bath was affirmed to me as being correct, thus encouraging me to throw myself wholeheartedly into the experience of being there.

Knowing I'd be without the Internet for some weeks, I'd compiled a folder of useful information that would enable me to continue my pursuits of dance and yoga, being the oil that moves my cogs *and* provides me with some work. I began to check out the local area and was delighted to discover a French café that had just opened prior to my arrival there, a fabulous butcher with excellent banter on tap, and an old-fashioned green grocer where the produce was grown locally. And then of course, there were many walks to discover. I had definitely found a spot that was ripe for some enjoyment.

It wasn't long before a couple of phone calls with the young man I'd met just before my move paved the way for his first visit to Bath, proving to be the first of many. It was at the end of his first weekend visit that I waved goodbye through the settling darkness from my third floor window that I recalled that exact same scene from a dream a few months earlier, right down

31

to the words that he spoke as he called up to me from the garden below - further confirmation that all was as it should be. So, the scene was set, but for what exactly?

I was poised to engage in what work I could procure, but it was months before anything came along. As I assumed my move was permanent, it seemed natural to try to earn a living. I hadn't considered that perhaps this was a time meant for another type of work, something beyond what I expected.

My network of friends led me to meet a lovely Irish medium with whom I struck up a friendship. She was keen to get to know me better but was puzzled as to why I'd moved there, despite her open-mindedness. A reading with her pointed me to the healing it seemed I needed to address; it was to do with the old Roman baths. I was used to the concept of healing issues from past lives, but I also knew that one doesn't have to physically visit such places in order to do so; that particular aspect still puzzles me. However, as soon as I left her house, I shot down to the Roman baths for a late afternoon reccy.

That weekend's visit from my man was indeed interesting and perhaps pivotal. We visited the Roman baths and were standing by the old steps to the temple of Minerva when two waves of intense energy washed over me. I had stood alone on that very spot only a few days before and yet nothing occurred then - perhaps it was something to do with our combined energies...?

The energetic waves left me feeling somewhat off balance and so we decided to return home, where I immediately lay down on my couch. Doing the work I do, I am used to observing how the physical body can be a conduit for all sorts of energy, and that we sometimes need another person to help us move and transmute that energy so that it doesn't impede our own natural flow. With this principle in mind and working entirely instinctively, I guided the hands of my partner to the places on my being where energy seemed to need releasing, despite him not having any prior experience of such work. Perhaps it was my obvious distress that moved him to stunned silence and compliance, but the releasing continued until I felt empty and still, with sleep coming soon after.

⌘

The next few months rumbled by happily as the relationship appeared to be moving forward, and love was definitely in the air. However, in the spring of the following year, this changed abruptly as the strain of long distance and poor communication caused a sudden, heart-rending break-up. The effect of the break-up was akin to the death of a loved one, such was the pain of my grief. The tears flowed; my life slowed almost to a standstill, and I felt I could no longer live in the place that had become ours. I made the difficult decision to let my flat go and put my furniture into storage, but the memories from my nine months that I lived in Bath will be treasured forever.

I was fortunate enough to be able to stay with my sister in Wiltshire while I tried to get my life back on track and decide on my next course of action. My sister and I had always got on well together when back home, although we'd since grown into who we are now - two strong individuals – and living under the same roof wasn't as easy as we thought. However, we muddled through and came out the other side intact; probably not an experience we will repeat but I was most grateful to have somewhere to stay. I often reflect upon the differences between siblings, even among my own boys, and how we all grow up and apart in ways that could not be perceived from knowing the youngsters.

Eventually, after several trips back to Hertfordshire, I decided to return to Tring, not least so that I could be more supportive to my boys. I was not entirely happy with how things were going with my eldest and wanted to be close by to give guidance and help as necessary. Plus, I had had the foresight to keep some of my old clients by running a monthly clinic in the area.

Procuring a house to rent in the area had become extremely difficult, especially from a distance. Every time I went to view a property, the previous viewer had snapped it up. It was the issue of distance that had me firstly rent a holiday cottage for a week, then to take up the offer of a room in a friend's cottage for a few weeks. The latter turned out to be rather interesting.

The day I moved into said cottage, my friend was away so her father let me in. At first sniff, my heart sank. It was a 'cat' house i.e. the cats went wherever they liked and one it seemed was not particularly healthy on the inside. It seemed a spot of cleaning was on the cards if I was going to stay there, so I got busy. Seven hours and much cleaning later, I was just about ready to settle in after buying new hair-free bedding and evicting the sources of some seriously evil smells.

A few days later, I helped move some stuff into the loft and clear some space in the front bedroom, thus disturbing some ancient dust and cat 'material'. A few days later, I began to have abdominal pain and developed a fever – I feared the invasion of something I really didn't want. Fortunately, following a prompt by my instinct, I had some ground clove capsules with me (often used in the treatment of parasites) and began to take those regularly; these seemed to help but only in the short term. I ordered some anti-parasitic herbs from a friend and engaged in what

35

needed to be done to tackle what I guessed to be the problem.

Not one to take the gift of accommodation lightly, I then spent several days bringing order to the over-grown back garden, dislodging all sorts of soil-based microbes in the process, be they plant or cat based. Of course, the physical activity was good, but I'd not realised how vulnerable I was as a result of the escalating stress levels eroding my immune system and how easily I fell prey to whatever foreign bodies were in the environment. It seemed that this issue would cause many more problems for me over the ensuing years.

⌘

It was during one of my return trips to Hertfordshire that I decided to pay a visit to my old dance haunt. Coincidentally, I bumped into my ex (the one who jilted me in Bath) who had no idea I'd be there. There was a moth to a flame moment; suffice to say it was emotional. Not long after the blue touch paper had been re-lit, we began to see each other again, although with some reserve. Despite the uncertainty of our relationship, my man nevertheless was instrumental in the process of me getting somewhere to live, for which I will always be grateful

By the time I was able move into my new home, I was extremely stressed and so ready to sink into my own space. Sadly, my man was a little too excited at being in my company again and only gave me one day alone before moving himself in. Whilst it was fun at first, it really wasn't what I needed. If I had been stronger, I would have taken a firmer stance and restored my own internal peace and released the stresses that had accumulated over the last year or so, but my energy and resistance were low, and I acceded to his wishes. A few weeks later, my eldest son moved back in with me. Observing how we all rubbed along was interesting, but not exactly peaceful. In fact, within two months of our cohabitation, severe cracks became apparent in the relationship and my man moved back out. The peace and ease I so desperately sought was not to be found for some time.

And so, as I moved through the next 12 months, there seemed to be one health issue after another, pretty much like a row of dominoes falling down. Oh, the symptoms were real enough, sometimes painful and often debilitating, but all tests proved nothing, except to be very puzzling and frustrating.

Looking back now, it was plain to see that my body was not having the chance it should have had to repair, and whichever system was the weakest was where the main problem would show up. My immune system was clearly not functioning well, and it seemed that every time I went out socially I would pick up some other infection, but there was still something I hadn't understood.

Whilst I was still trying to work the basis of my situation out, I began to rebuild my immune system, so that I could feel up to working again, and this is how I worked out my recovery:

Garlic was absolutely <u>the best</u> to zap all bugs and viruses in my body. 1-3 cloves, finely chopped and placed in a finger depth of water, swished around and downed in one! It's powerful stuff and can give a feeling of nausea on an empty stomach, so I generally ate breakfast straight after. The active ingredient – allicin – is reported to remain active within the body for around 60 hours, but I found it knocked out the effect of other supplements, so I always took it alone. I also found that once it began to sprout, the garlic wasn't as effective.

Monolaurin, derived from coconut, was significant in recovering my immunity from a gut level (I used **Lauricidin** pellets, although omitted to read the label which read 'Do not chew', and once sprinkled some onto my muesli – it was like eating soap!). After 2 months of Lauricidin, I switched to an increased amount of coconoil throughout the day. Also, use of probiotics - mostly **Saccharomyces Boulardii** - cycled with **Optibac for every day** as needed, was helpful. For some reason these two don't work together, a factor I also found common among other supplements, so it's not as simple as chucking a handful of capsules into your mouth and assuming you'll flourish. The Saccharomyces Boulardii was great for tackling candida overgrowth (due to antibiotics) but the Optibac seems to balance other flora.

While my lymphatic system needed boosting, several superficial lymph nodes were tender so I resumed my old practice of jumping on my **rebounder** to ease the stagnant feeling I had. This, coupled with daily brisk walks of 20-40 minutes, depending upon available energy, kept my energy relatively steady (activity helps to ease liver congestion, especially in the morning).

As my toxic load had been high for some time, I had to be careful about the healing protocol I employed in order to avoid further overload. Every cleansing action increased the level of toxins in the blood for a while, so if the load was too great, I'd feel like I had a massive hangover, and indeed, this did happen a few times. I mostly used **Ornithine** and **Deactivated Charcoal** between meals to counter this, but also **Plant Source Antioxidants** (with milk thistle) to ease my burgeoning liver. I would know if I needed the latter as I'd find it difficult to get to sleep, despite being dog-tired. (Another remedy I used for being unable to get to sleep was Bupleurum tincture, a Chinese remedy, which worked well).

All of the above was good and helped me begin the trek back to better health, but I knew I *still* had to find the root cause of what I was beginning to see had been a repetitive cycle in my life since my teens.

One day, I looked out a **genomic profile** about my personal detox ability from Genova Diagnostics at **https://www.gdx.net/uk/** that I'd had done at a seminar back in 2003 which highlighted a possible problem with **methylation** and began to research the subject.   I   discovered   the   website **www.enzymestuff.com**; although aimed primarily at supporting those in the autistic spectrum, I found it to be highly informative in putting together many snippets of information that I'd previously known were relevant but hadn't understood the significance of in the wider picture. I cross-referenced this information with the writings of Dr Sarah Myhill upon the subject – **www.drmyhill.co.uk**, and some of the writings of Walter Last at **www.health-science-spirit.com.** The sum of what I found was most interesting.

Methylation is a term for the addition or removal of a methyl group (a methyl group is made up of one carbon connected to three hydrogen atoms) to a compound or element. The joining of a methyl group to an element or compound in the human body can begin a process, such as activating an enzyme or turning on a gene, whereas the removal of the methyl group can stop a process. Hundreds of these types of reactions occur naturally in the human body every day when all the components are present.

Although there are hundreds of methyl reactions in the body, several key points stood out for me:

- 'Getting' methyl groups turns on **detox reactions** in the body, helping it be rid of chemicals, including phenols.

- 'Getting' methyl groups turns on serotonin, and thus melatonin, production. This means that if I am an under-methylator and choose to increase my methylation (via food or supplementation), I could improve my levels of serotonin and melatonin, thus improving sleep potential.

- Excess niacin (B3) is metabolized by methylation, thus using up methyl groups (useful for over-methylators).

So how would I go about improving my natural detox processes, lighten the load of my burgeoning liver and ultimately increase my energy levels?

Well, I'd started down this route already by reaching for some HCl (Betaine Hydrochloride), something that I'd been directed to use as part of the metabolic typing program some years before. However, I was still supplementing on a day-to-day basis, simply by dowsing what I was drawn to from my cupboard. Whilst this seemed to be working, I didn't have a real framework or understanding of what was actually happening until later.

The methylation section on **www.ensymestuff.com** points out how deficiencies prevail in many people, thus affecting whether some of the methylation reactions actually occur. So, along with the HCl, I began to supplement zinc and B12, B6 (as P-5-P) and folate from leafy vegetables. I already knew I'd been very low in zinc for some time as I had hardly any sense of taste or smell.

It seems the trick, as with most things, is to find the balance. Too many methyl groups running around the body, which can sometimes be a source of aggression or agitation, can be tackled by taking Niacin (B3), the processing of which *uses up* methyl groups. (I was told I was B3 deficient some years ago when tested on a NES machine, which surprised me at the time.)

Apparently, low levels of methyl groups in the body can lead to raised histamine levels (histadelia). This can make such a person overly sensitive to foods that are high in salicylates or phenols, which are common in foods we might regard as tasty. As I consider this viewpoint, I recall how I once ended up in hospital with an extreme histamine reaction, despite never having had any allergic symptoms before.

Now, when I consider my highly sensitive nature in context of the above picture, whereby I potentially accumulate stress easily, and now knowing that *stress* is one of the factors that can *turn off* methylation, it becomes easier to get the bigger picture of why my health has been so variable for so long and reinstates my hope of achieving consistently better energy levels that I should have access to when I learn how to notice how the biochemical cycles feel. So now I observe my attractions or aversions to certain foods and drinks and humour my instinct because it's generally correct, whatever the reason.

What else did I learn at this time?

It has taken long term, consistent efforts to move through this phase, working not just on the physical aspects of my health, but also my mental and emotional outlook. Fortunately, I have a dogged determination to learn from all of my experiences and to come out the other side stronger and wiser.

Something that seemed extremely important to my recovery, perhaps due to my sensitivity, was **sleeping alone**. It seemed if I was to recharge fully with no interference to my aura, having the bed to myself was and still is essential (since childhood I've always hated sharing a bed). Similarly, when I awake even now, I like to stay 'within' as I return to my conscious world; I quietly feel my way into the day in my own way, checking my internal monitors and working out what I'm feeling today, not perhaps in the way that another might want or expect (this too has been the case all of my life). I guess this kind of preference doesn't fit many peoples' idea of a relationship, but these days I know I must consider myself first.

I continue to explore other options to support the work of the liver even now, as I feel there are still aspects of function that I must work out if I am to function without feeling like the brakes are on all of the time.

Meaningful relationships

It is my belief that the biggest influence in anyone's life is the relationship between them and their parents. The first seven years of life reportedly involve downloading and copying all interrelations from parent to child, thus forming a master program, and as such forms the behavioural conditioning that lies atop the blueprint of each and every one of us.

As the child moves towards and into adulthood, the circle of influence widens, but the interpretation of life's new relationships is still subconsciously governed by the early programming. The influence of that first conditioning continues to affect subsequent relationships in our lives until such a time as we question its viability and choose to amend the program. As relationships may well be one of the biggest stressors in our life, it really is helpful to put them into the context of our in-built filters and ask the kind of questions that ultimately create change within our self.

As a highly sensitive being, born during what I perceived were times of high stress (my most significant memory), I became used to running on adrenaline from an early age. This, coupled with a deep-seated need for privacy and time alone, meant that my life was an emotional roller coaster - from being startled, over-excited or angry to being completely exhausted. The effects became evident via frequent bouts of low blood sugar and therefore an inability to concentrate or perform well throughout my school years. I remember the joy of competing in sports, only to feel my energy quickly fade as I my blood sugar dropped. I remember the long walk up the lane from the school bus to home, feeling I barely had enough energy to put one foot in front of the other. I feel sad when I think back on my school years, as I know I could have achieved so much more had there been someone looking out for me.

It is not hard to work out that such grounding meant I had little understanding of how balance or stability felt, let alone self-love, and how later I might be able to achieve that for myself. That took half a century to build. In the meantime, I dove through years of 'trial-and-error' relationships within work, personal life and of course family, each bringing its own mixture of trouble, strife and just enough delight to keep me going.

My inherent interest in people and how we relate to each other led me to continually seek yet more answers to the ever-present question of 'Why' that characteristically dominates my mind. It was only when a friend introduced me to Human Design that clarity emerged, many Why's were answered and I gained some of that elusive *knowing*. It didn't necessarily change how I relate to certain people, but at least now I can understand some of why we interact the way we do, so I don't waste time or energy stressing about it.

Why do I mention any of this? Well, perhaps because I'm so sensitive, various relationships have had an adverse effect upon my health, but along the way, I embraced many life lessons, so that now, I make much better choices about what is right for my journey ahead.

I have learned that relationships are the biggest investment we make in life, and yes, they can be risky, exasperating, stressful or joyous, but they are *so* much more. Relationships are the vehicle by which I learn about myself as I dive ever deeper into life and investigate my own true potential. That was and continues to be the case today.

Balancing Act ~ being an HSP

During the last two years, I've come to realise, via the work of my good friend Gitte Lassen in Iceland, that I am a **H**ighly **S**ensitive **P**erson. I didn't even realise that research had been done to highlight such a group of people; I thought everyone had the potential to sense things in the way that I do. In light of this information, I've been able to look at the bigger picture of my life and see how and why stress has affected me more intensely than some.

Because stress is a subjective thing, i.e. the intensity of it is determined by ones' own sensitivity, it seemed that my biochemistry suffered big time, hence a string of mystery health issues appeared over recent years that highlighted my predicament and pre-empted my need to work on strategies that would enable me to deal with it. Whilst I've done plenty of research into my own biochemistry in order to get back to good health, the most difficult aspect of this sensitivity was to develop the emotional resilience that I lacked, being one of the main sources of my high stress levels. One of the tools I've used over the last 20 years to help me understand my energy flow is **Biorhythms;** I find it a useful indicator of how much energy I can expect on a day-to-day basis. (You can see more about this in the A-Z.) More importantly, understanding that when the three main biorhythms – physical, emotional and intellectual - are all low, one can feel totally exhausted for a week with poor digestion and disrupted sleep. At such times, it is important to nurture oneself more so rather than resort to stimulants, and get more rest in order to be ready for the inevitable upswing in energy as the biorhythms rise again – the little used word 'acceptance' being apt here.

Another thing I do is keep an ear to the ground regarding any planetary activity that may affect my energy, or that of anyone I'm working with. I generally check up on such things if I notice persistent behaviour or symptoms that are out of character or common amongst various individuals.

More recently, I've been using **pressure points** that send energy through the meridians of the body, and have been duly surprised at how helpful this was on many occasions to balance not just the physical, but also emotional disturbances that upset the general flow of energy throughout my body. On numerous occasions, this energetic shift has led to an increase in wellbeing. Some of the pressure points are the same as those used in **EFT** tapping (Emotional Freedom Technique), whilst others are from the teachings of Donna Eden.

On the physical side, I found that for me, frequent strong activity is required to generate a steady flow of energy throughout the body - the kind of energy surge that releases endorphins, improves confidence and frees up space in the liver, thus having a balancing effect upon the whole day. If this is not possible, then I may do some breathing exercises, for without an energy flow, stagnation quickly occurs, both mentally and physically. So activity needs to be regular if momentum is to be achieved and maintained – more so with advancing age I find.

The above activities are conscious and require forward thinking until new habits are formed. I, like most people, operate a good deal of the time from my subconscious, so the effort of conscious thinking can be tiring. However, with consistent application and willpower, I manage to stay focused enough to enforce good habits most of the time! During times of learning new ways of being, I find it is important to expend energy wisely, only committing to what is needed, rather than thoughtlessly frittering away precious energy where there is little or no return. That way, the new ways of doing things can be achieved much more quickly. Frivolous times can and will return once a new course has been set.

In times of high stress, herbs like **Rhodiola** are invaluable to help balance the biochemistry of the body. **Phosphatidylserine** is useful for mopping up an excess of cortisol that can occur as a result of prolonged stress; the first signs of this for me are a sort of tightness in the brain; too much cortisol can perpetuate the feeling of stress as well as prevent restful sleep (not to mention the many other effects of excess cortisol). So you see how important breaking the biochemical effects of stress is, just as the ability to listen well to the needs of the body and offer whatever support it needs *in the moment* is also necessary.

To sum up, maintaining a conscious approach for long enough to switch the habitual patterns that once existed for some that are more appropriate for my current goal is crucial in order to walk the path of my potential

Balancing Act Flow Chart

This chart depicts in simplified terms a summary of how I've come to view my personal operating system, what affects it and how.

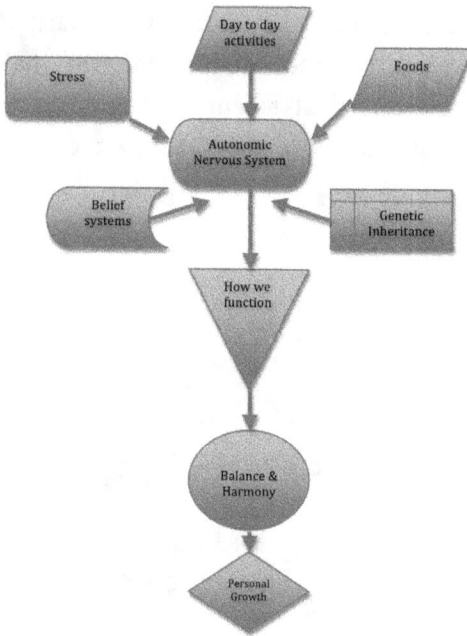

Autonomic Nervous System (ANS)

I learned a lot about the autonomic nervous system when I became a Metabolic Typing Advisor, but here is a potted version.

This part of the nervous system regulates the activities of smooth muscle, cardiac muscle, and certain glands, all without conscious control. Its name came about because scientists thought it operated independently of the Central Nervous System, but that was found to be untrue. It is regulated by the cerebral cortex, hypothalamus and medulla oblongata.

Some of the automatic activities of the Autonomic Nervous System (ANS) are changes in pupil size, blood vessel dilation, adjustment of heartbeat, sphincter control, rate of peristalsis and secretion of most glands.

There are two branches to the ANS – **sympathetic** and **parasympathetic**. Many body parts have connections to both branches; one branch *stimulates* and the other *decreases* activity. In simplified terms, the sympathetic branch prepares the body for 'fight or flight' and the parasympathetic branch for 'rest and digest'. Our genetic inheritance and how those genes are being expressed will dictate how our ANS *normally* functions within us and so provides a benchmark, and when we function at that part of the ANS scale, we will feel at our best. However, there are many factors that can and do affect normal functioning.

Because the ANS affects the metabolic rate, and the metabolic rate affects the ANS, we begin to understand how food choices can create a see-sawing of the ANS, either speeding it up or slowing it down, both of which may affect our sense of wellbeing. So, whilst the ANS is not as important as the heart in the greater scheme of things, it is at the heart of creating balance.

What affects ANS function?

Genetic Inheritance

How our ANS functions is mostly rooted in our genes but not totally, for there is much we can be exposed to, or choose to do that can affect how those genes are expressed. The latter is explored in a branch of science called Epigenetics.

Foods

The main food groups, known as macronutrients, are carbohydrate, fat and protein. Most of us are familiar with the idea of consuming a balanced ratio of foods from each of these groups regularly every day (that idea would certainly have filtered down through many families from the post-war era into the subsequent generation, but probably became diluted in the last decade or so.)

Now, it is posited that wherever our genes place us on the ANS scale, we will realise a feeling of wellbeing by consuming the appropriate ratio of each macronutrient group for that part of the scale. However, the mixed messages that modern adulterated foods give our bodies confuse and interfere with our biochemistry, creating cravings and disrupting normal function and flow. So it's not just about having an eating routine, but being discerning about *what* we eat if we are to become more conscious of the long term effect upon our own wellbeing.

Day to day activities
Eating, working, playing, sleeping, and environment are the active aspects of what can affect the ANS, either positively or negatively.

Belief Systems
Belief systems are the passive aspect of what affects our ANS. We inherit some belief systems during our formative years of living with our carers, and we adopt others along the way, but they all tend to give rise to expectations. Whether or not those expectations are met can dictate how we react/respond and therefore what emotions come into play.

Stress
How we each perceive stress is dependent upon the extent of our own sensitivity, and thus how we interpret each direct experience. Stress can build up because of how we emotionally respond (coloured by our inherent belief systems), so it is not fixed and can be changed. How we tend to release stress is a personal thing, but it does need releasing if an excessive outburst is to be avoided. Massage, laughing, dancing and music therapy have all been

shown to reduce the high levels of cortisol produced by stress.

Balance & Harmony

For me, balance and harmony is something I have to work at constantly. How much I 'try' may seem contradictory to what I'm trying to achieve, but I've not yet learned the easy way – I'm still practicing. I use the silence, meditation, nature, exercise and the other tools mentioned in this book. Without those things, I soon fall back into either reacting to life or stagnating within it. I think and feel better when balanced and that's all I'm seeking.

Personal Growth

Growth is a personal choice; not everyone wants to do it. In my opinion, it's what I'm here for. I have a desire to meet my potential, to be everything I can possibly be and to reach the end of this life feeling satisfied that I have done all I can to help myself and others be all that they can be.

PART II

My Toolbox

This chapter is made up of the essentials that have become my toolbox for monitoring and maintaining my health and wellbeing on a day-to-day basis. It has to be said that I find dowsing an incredibly useful tool, so it is no wonder that I place it at the top of my list of useful tools and recommend anyone and everyone to learn how to do it for themselves. However, I also check my biorhythms on a daily basis to check what I can expect in terms of energy levels. I use http://www.biorhythmonline.com you can read more in the A-Z of Resources.

Dowsing

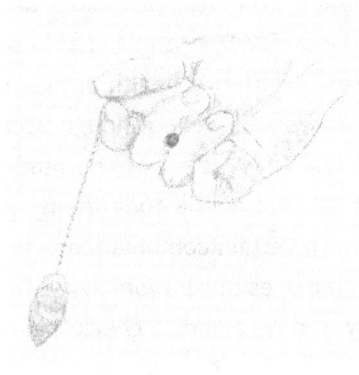

I first came across dowsing back in the 1980's via a retired teacher, David Perry, who'd been exploring earth energies for some time. He'd worked extensively around the UK to help relieve many people's homes of geopathic stress, which is a type of earth energy that can undermine sleep and health. When on-site, he'd use a pair of telescopic car aerials (as they fitted into his pocket) which were bent into an 'L' shape in order to locate the 'grid' lines, before inserting copper pipes into the ground (some call this earth acupuncture) in order to divert the geopathic stress that was affecting the home he was working on. He helped many people recover normal sleep patterns and improve health issues as far ranging as epilepsy and cancer by doing this. When working at home, he'd use a pendulum over a floor plan to ascertain the same information and then visit the property later.

The thing that interested me about another aspect of his accomplished dowsing ability was that he would use a pendulum to dowse food charts in order to help people who were suffering health or dietary issues. In the main, this worked well, although accurate at the time, it was limited in effect as the readings he took only related to the time he took them, not in an on-going basis or in certain combinations. In light of this information, it makes much more sense for individuals to learn how to dowse and to check their readings for themselves, in order to cope with ever changing circumstances and biochemistry.

So, in these complicated times, when you need to quickly find out what is best for you in the here and now, dowsing can be a really useful tool that neatly side-steps your conscious mind to draw answers from your Higher Self, or what T.C. Lethbridge once termed the Super Conscious. Dowser Neil Stiller of www.area9.info terms this need as a *Quest*, because you are seeking something – the answer to a question, the location of an object, or a direction to take, and it should be of pure intent and without personal gain.

To begin, buy or make a pendulum – a small stone or weight can be attached to a 15-20cm (6-10") chain or thin cord, providing enough weight to hold the cord/chain taught and swing from a balanced point. Yes, it's even possible to make a pendulum with a piece of chewing gum on the end of a piece of cotton! You can buy fancy pendulums from crystal shops, although some may be light in weight, just find one that you feel happy with. A long string or cord is more sensitive to small muscular movements but takes longer to complete a movement than a short string. When starting, a long string may be best, switching to a shorter length as you become more accomplished.

A lightweight pendulum needs less energy to respond but is easily swayed by the wind if outdoors. These factors should be considered when you're 'tuning' your pendulum.

According to Neil Stiller, an easy way to 'tune' your pendulum is to hold the string in your non-dominant hand, between the thumb and index finger, and hold the upward facing palm of your dominant hand under the pendulum without touching. Start by holding the cord about 2 inches away from the pendulum and slowly let out more cord to determine the point at which the pendulum assumes a healthy swing. That will be the best length for you. If you are sensitive, your pendulum may make very large circles all the time when using this length; if this is so, then use the shorter length – the point at which your pendulum first started to move. Mark this 'holding point' by making a knot in the string.

Getting started

You'll need to 'program' your pendulum i.e. ascertain how it wishes to show you a 'Yes' or 'No' answer. Look at your own mindset and how you ask questions. Initially you may get answers from your subconscious mind, but over time you will know when this is happening by knowing yourself better. When you work with your pendulum, the questions need to be 'closed' i.e. answered with a 'Yes' or 'No' *and* unambiguous. As you begin, resist the temptation to *make* the pendulum move – when your intention is clear, the pendulum will swing of its own accord, this can be a forwards and back swing (or leading edge) or a circular motion.

By itself your pendulum has no magical abilities; it is a tool. All it does is to amplify the input that is channelled (sometimes from a spirit/energetic source) through your higher self, helping you attain clear answers to your questions. As with all tools, you must take care of your pendulum so that it is clean and in good condition when needed.

When you first begin, you may get 101 different answers to the same basic questions. Don't be put off, this is merely an indication of how you're still getting used to being mentally neutral. The main thing is to dowse with total detachment. Consistent practice is essential. You will not become skilled overnight; it can take many months or years.

There are numerous books that teach this art, and it may take a great deal of practice before you can totally trust the outcome, but in time, you'll be able to 'feel' the accuracy of your dowsing and expand the subject material that you dowse to anything you need clarification upon such as food, supplements or actions. Neil Stiller's site – www.area9.info gives lots of extra information upon dowsing, and, if you're keen to have tuition, he also runs workshops.

Health History
However we are born and into whatever circumstances, we can all become adept at creating distractions that neatly sidestep that which our instinct

would have us do and learn important lessons from. One such distraction is the very human art of forgetting. It may well be a clever subconscious mind that on the one hand has us forget to take a vitamin pill that the physical form no longer needs, or it may be the mind creating a diversion in order to avoid something that makes us feel uncomfortable. The mind can be very skilled in avoiding tactics but either way, how much of forgetting is to dismiss something temporarily or to avoid it completely?

So why mention the forgetting skill? Well, it seems to me that if we are to learn from previous experiences, it is necessary for us to remember the salient parts of the journey, be it to do with health or emotions, so that we know what to do in a similar scenario. By that I mean to remember the lessons learned, how we felt, that it was finite and that life did indeed go on. I suspect that in my young life, it may have appeared to others that I was over-dramatising what I went through at times, but that's not the case, it's just that there was no yard stick by which to gauge the experience, so *it was big*! If the same experience were to play out a year later, I would automatically remember the similarity, and the effect would be reduced according to how well I dealt with it at the time.

In order to allay poor memory and to document a growing list of symptoms, in my 30's, I started to write a potted health history to make it a reference for whomever I sought help from, in order to help make an accurate diagnosis by supplying as much relevant information as possible. It's also rather difficult to cite ailments when you're not feeling well; things inevitably get missed. Keeping a record of ailments and changes was a good starting point that I could later pull out and amend as necessary and has formed the backbone of *my* own research journey.

Writing a treatment plan

When we go to the doctors, we are often issued with a prescription and then told to return if the problem persists, sometimes with only a vague idea of what to expect, mainly because we've been given a broad-spectrum medicine with an approximation of how it will behave in *our* bodies.

Instead of the haphazard approach of trying a few 'off-the-peg' supplements, I broadened my thinking into making my own treatment plan, using my pendulum to work out the details. The questions I posed were:

- ❖ **what to take** – my symptoms would dictate the general direction then some research would highlight the specifics.

- ❖ **how much to take** – amounts vary and are not always what we assume, but depend on current biochemistry. Factors to consider are current level of toxicity (always present in any illness), hormonal levels, the ability to maintain homeostatic balance, functional requirements (the need to work) and sleeping ability.

- ❖ **when** - best time of day, with or without food, alone or with something else, and **for how long** before reviewing.

This approach even applies to taking garlic, which I found cancels out the action of many other supplements for up to 60 hours, but is a fabulous antibiotic. I keep experiential notes during a treatment plan then modify as necessary, but the key is to assess the journey and how it made me feel for future reference, so I quickly know what works for when I need it in future. However, I would still dowse the situation each day to take into consideration the changing biochemistry. Below is an example of how I might note things down.

What to take	How much	When	How often	How I felt
Raw garlic	1 clove	Before breakfast	Alternate days	Brighter, more energy, and clear thinking after just 30 mins. Lasted 24 hrs
De-activated Charcoal	2 capsules	Between meals, as necessary	When head aches, due to increased toxic load	Headache went within 20 mins; thinking clear.

Medicine/supplement cupboard

Most people have a cupboard in their home, where they keep off-the-shelf pharmaceuticals, sticking plasters and TCP in readiness for life's little disasters. What we keep as our medicines usually starts as a continuation of what our parents used on us, then as we learn and evolve, the contents will change to something different according to our own trials and experiences until we have a support system that's based upon what we believe works best for us.

The above has certainly been true for me and I now have my own mini apothecary for me and mine. Some items come and go, according to short-term needs, whilst others fall into the categories of aromatherapy, herbals or homeopathy, being formulations that I have tried and tested over time and can vouch for their efficacy as a repeatable process.

My approach has always been to spot a potential problem early on and nip it in the bud, before it can become serious. This has worked well for several decades, including bringing up two children who hardly ever saw a doctor. Knowing myself well enough to spot when something doesn't feel right is the first step. Observing the situation just long enough to see its picture, then dowsing for the right remedy is what follows.

Key essentials:

Mini-homeopathic kit; although in constant use whilst my children were growing up, I tend to use it only occasionally now, perhaps for the Arnica.

Throat: Internally, salt water gargle, repeating until eased.

Eternally: Various essential oils, as listed below.

Thyroid/Metabolism: Lugol's iodine: 1-2 drops in water (see A-Z for further info)

Immune system: Thymotrate, Zinc, Vitamin D over winter.

Blood: Ornithine, Deactivated charcoal.

Energy: Magnesium, taken with Malic Acid as needed.

Digestion: HCl & Pepsin, Pancreatin/lipase.

Methylation: Niacin, Vitamin B6, B12, MSM.

Hormones:

Pregnenolone: as needed) *in line*

Evening Primrose oil   ) *with normal cycle*

Progesterone   ) *as above.*

Maca root

Gut: Candida Support (Saccharomyces Boulardii), Optibac Daily; these two don't seem to work together.

Liver: Plant Source Antioxidants with Milk Thistle, Burdock root.

Stress: Rhodiola: liquid is faster acting than capsules and easier to tailor the amount, but each have their place.

Phosphatidyl Serine – to mop up the excess Cortisol produced in times of stress.

Emotions: Bach Flower Remedies – various, according to needs at the time.

Essential Oils
Essential oils have been my friends for decades, with many favoured recommendations coming from Maggie Tisserand back in the 90's. I have found over the years that, as with supplements, not all the oils you can buy are equal in their effectiveness, so it pays to invest in high quality oils for good results and to store them correctly to promote longevity. Whilst the more common ones are available on the high street, some of the ones mentioned below would have to be ordered.

Arnica – usually sold as a blended oil for topical treatment of bruising.

Lavender – the one never to be without. A few drops on the pillows of my children helped them settle and sleep well. Can be used neat over the throat/ glands to stem soreness. I sometimes apply it neat to neck or lower back if feeling 'off colour' before getting into a bath, as the hot water helps it penetrate more readily.

It's also *The Best* for treating burns, and if used immediately, can avoid the skin peeling off. This I can testify to!

Ravensara – this anti-viral/antibacterial oil is my preference above Tea Tree, and is reportedly 10 times more effective, yet has a pleasing mild smell.

Red Thyme - an excellent oil for fungal nail problems or verrucas – a condition that is easy to pick up from others, but not so easy to get rid of. Persistence pays off; rub neat oil into the affected area every day until improvement is seen. Again, a very strong oil, but used with care is a good alternative to allopathic solutions. Alternatively, you can use Iodine.

Recipes

Concentration blend

Blend together equal amounts of the essential oils **Basil, Rosemary and Grapefruit.** Add a few drops of the mix to a tissue to sniff or place in a vaporiser to aid concentration. This works especially well for exams or interviews when combined with **Rhodiola** to combat the nerves.

Elderberry & Peppermint Compound

Years ago, I used to buy this, but for some time have been unable to find it, so decided to formulate my own recipe – it's just as I remember but nicer.

Ingredients

4 pints of Elderberries – equates to a carrier bag full of

berry clusters

3/4 pint boiling water

8 oz light brown sugar

1/4 tsp ground cinnamon

1/4 tsp ground allspice

Essential oils of Peppermint (15 drops), Cardomom

(8 drops) and Ravensara (6 drops)

1. Place all the berries, still upon their stalks, in a large bowl and cover with water to which

you've added a few drops of iodine. This should bring out all resident spiders and earwigs!

2. Drain, and (wearing rubber gloves), gently 'rub' the berries off their branches into a large mixing bowl.

3. Meanwhile, in a pan, simmer the water, sugar and spices together, ready to pour over the prepared berries.

4. Cover and place keep in the fridge for 48 hrs to macerate.

5. After the 48 hrs, strain off the liquid, pressing the berries with the back of a ladle, and discard the berries. I got just over a pint of liquid concentrate.

6. Heat gently to 65 degrees c, then cool down to 35 degrees before adding the essential oils. Still well for several minutes to distribute the oils.

7. Pour into sterile glass bottles – this quantity fills 4 x 250ml bottles.

To use, place 1 tablespoon of mixture into a mug and top up with hot water. Smell, sip and enjoy! This mixture can be used to treat coughs and colds, or used to stave them off.

Four Robbers blend

Having used the 'official' version of this oil and been impressed by its potency, I searched for a suitable recipe online to make my own and this is what I found:

Take the following essential oils -

> 40 drops Clove Bud
>
> 36 drops Lemon
>
> 20 drops Cinnamon Bark
>
> 16 drops Eucalyptus
>
> 10 drops Rosemary.

Add all to a dark glass bottle, shake well and store in a cool place, away from sunlight.

In my experience, viruses are expert at hiding in the dense tissue surrounding the spine until such a time as energy or immunity is low, then they seize their opportunity to flourish; this is when the Four Robbers blend comes into its own. I have found initial symptoms to be a persistent dull ache at either the back of the neck or the lower back/sacral area, so I usually dribble some of the oil blend down my spine or just rub it into the affected area. NB: this oil blend can feel like it's burning at first so I would dilute the blend with a little plain base oil. Also it can stain clothes, so I ensure it's rubbed in well. If caught early enough, this mixture can stave off an illness.

Oral panacea

Get a small glass jar and pour in about a tablespoon of clear honey, then add 6 drops of Ravensara (3-4 drops for children) and stir with a skewer or similar. Leave to stand for a few hours if possible. I take quarter of a teaspoon every few hours until the symptoms decrease. This can be used at the first signs of a sore throat to stave off a worsening problem, or a virus that's emerged and needs to be checked internally. I used this many times on my children for sore throats, in order to nip infection in the bud. Children tend to respond quickly so don't need many doses, but use your discretion.

Treatment for Thrush

Thrush essentially comes from an overgrowth of candida in the gut (as well as being transmitted sexually), so it's quickest to treat both inside and out. During the treatment phase, remove coffee and alcohol from the diet as they raise the blood sugar significantly and are counterproductive to the treatment. This recipe is suitable for mild cases.

Internally – you will need to dowse the correct dosage for yourself, but as a guideline, 8 drops of tincture of myrrh in half a cup of water, taken 3 times a day on an empty stomach, for 3 days, is about right.

Douche – 5 drops of tincture of myrrh, 3 drops of lavender essential oil and half a teaspoon of coconoil in a quarter pint of warm water. Use this once a day for the 3 days.

Useful Plants

Garlic is always on standby (not sprouting) for tackling viral infections. At the onset of any viral or bacterial infection – or even just feeling slightly unwell, take 1-2 cloves of finely chopped garlic in 2 fingers of water just before breakfast. Yes, the odour can be a problem, but by eating parsley and drinking parsley tea (which is also rich in calcium), that issue can be lessened significantly. Repeat as necessary.

I keep a regularly trimmed **dandelion** plant in the garden as a general digestive tonic; eat the younger leaves that have only been in partial sun – full sun and overgrowth makes them bitter. I also keep **sage** (good as a hormone balancer) and **lemon balm** (calming) in the garden to make infusions.

Other Considerations

It is worth noting at this point that there are several conditions that will always undermine a return to good health whilst they are allowed to affect the body; heavy metal toxicity (i.e. mercury), geopathic stress, a parasitic overgrowth (we all carry parasites to some extent), and a leaky gut (from candida overgrowth).

The repetitive signals that any of the above could be present are when no matter what steps are taken to regain health, there always seems to be a back-sliding to lowered immunity, hormonal swings, poor temperature control, frequently low energy levels and of course the inevitable effects upon mood.

As a rule of thumb, whenever the body is under duress, it's best to avoid sugars, alcohol, refined carbohydrates and to limit fats, as doing so will generally mean a quicker return to a more balanced state, but this is only a short term measure.

Since the retention of toxic substances in the body is a great contributor to disease, the use of aluminium and non-stick cooking utensils should be avoided, stainless steel being a far better option.

In Summary

In this day and age, where information is readily available on any and every subject you could choose, there is no need for anyone to ignore the messages from their body that indicate the onset of a problem. The ultimate aim is to respond to the *earliest* signs from the body that something is amiss and do something about it, rather than waiting for someone else, who really doesn't know all the 'ins and outs' of your body or your life to tell you.

If you sit down and work out the chain of events that helped you arrive at the situation you're in, you can usually see the reason for any imbalance, and sometimes the solution too. Don't succumb to feelings of helplessness here, imagining it's a vast subject – that's what people who are usually trying to sell you something would have you believe. You will instinctively know from the events in your life what has led you to this point and roughly the direction to look in for the answers, so give it a go.

Sure, we can all procrastinate or avoid the actions of nurturing ourselves – usually this lack of action is rooted in a desire to be taken care of or rescued that still plays out from the broken record of our childhood – but this *can* be changed by conscious intention, and the good feeling that comes on the back of that is one that can be built upon.

Given the right foods and environment, the body is a self-regulating, self-healing, self-contained organism.

Finding Information to Trust

I am by nature a curious person, whose favourite question is 'why'. This means that I am always on the lookout for information that has a ring of truth that gives at least a starting point for further research. I find that I naturally filter out what doesn't hold true for me, and the things that I do resonate with I remember with ease, going back to look up more information from that source again and again. One such website that has been enormously helpful for me over recent years is that of Walter Last: www.health-science-spirit.com. Walter is a naturopath and a prolific writer for Nexus magazine over many years, as well as publishing his own books on all matters of health and healing. I find his writings to be very down to earth and practical so they resonate strongly with me.

Finding the right information is about being open and following only what feels right in this moment. It's like a trail of breadcrumbs, whereby whatever has resonance will lead the way to the correct information for my situation at that particular time. As time goes by, the required information may need to be more in-depth, or come from another source in order to deal with the changes that may have developed in my circumstances or biochemistry. Whatever the case, it's all about expanding the perspective and continuing to evolve with the confidence of additional knowledge. So instead of seeing the ever-changing journey as a confused mass of information, I learned to trust my instinct and only follow what or who resonates the most strongly with me.

PART III

A-Z of Resources

A

Acid/Alkaline – there is much information out there about the pro's and cons of being too much of either one, but here's the essence of what I've learned:

Our genetic make-up determines how our **Autonomic Nervous System (ANS)** functions – whether it's towards the sympathetic, para-sympathetic or balanced (somewhere between the two). Apparently, if ones' ANS operates predominantly from the sympathetic branch, one will be naturally acidic, and therefore needs to eat foods that are more alkaline to create balance and wellbeing.

If one's ANS operates predominantly from the para-sympathetic branch, one is naturally alkaline and will need to eat more protein, high purine foods to slow them down to a balanced state. Either way, your 'normal' acid/alkali state is pre-determined, but on top of that, what you consume determines how well you achieve balance over time and therefore how well you feel and perform.

How this translates is that some foods (and drinks) make you feel brighter and some foods dull your senses because of their effect on the ANS. For instance, grain-based drinks, like whisky or gin make me sleepy, whereas wine is fine. Knowing this can be handy if sleep won't come, but I have observed myself using this mechanism on occasion as a viable distraction to something I didn't want to do.

Being *too* acidic, or *too* alkaline show very similar symptoms, but mainly a lack of energy. The main way to tell if you've shifted from one state to another is that you suddenly have very different desires about which food groups you seek, and all sorts of abnormal cravings crop up as your internal barometer swings wildly. The quickest way to tell which direction to go in is to first try an alkaline piece of fruit such as orange, and then observe closely how it makes you feel. Then, eat a piece of meat and again observe. One food will make you feel good, one will make you feel worse - you'll have the answer within minutes, so you'll conclusively know which type of food you need more of. Read around the subject of Metabolic Typing for more clues and then try some experimenting of your own.

Action – we may be well read, but thinking is not the same thing as doing. Thought is head-based but does not bring knowledge. The body needs to be fed new actions that it can incorporate into its being in order to arrive at knowledge. The body is an experiential mechanism with inbuilt wisdom, but we can still add to that wisdom by gaining extra *knowing*. Make it a priority to DO a positive action on a regular basis; if you like it, keep repeating that action as appropriate until it has an aspect of becoming automated (anything that is not done regularly can and will be forgotten – it's part of being human). What you are looking to achieve, is the ability to get out of your own way and make some sort of investment in yourself without further distraction or judgment.

Adrenal glands – sit on top of each kidney and regulate many systems of the body, including our fight or flight responses. With frequent over stimulation, such as long term stress, the adrenals become exhausted and unable to contribute adequately or effectively to balancing the systems of the body. Adrenal exhaustion can have a knock on effect on the thyroid, thus slowing the metabolism. "The Cortisol Connection" by Shawn M Talbott explains this process and further information can be found at **www.thyroiduk.org.uk**. I have found some supplements, containing bovine adrenal concentrate, to be useful in strengthening these important glands and balancing my system as a whole, although returning to full power requires an approach that encompasses diet and lifestyle at the same time.

Affirmations – Since I first encountered affirmations many years ago, I was a tad sceptical – after all, how can uttering a few words over and over really change anything? Well over the years, it's become clear that uttering a few words here and there can have an effect, but only when you really mean what you say at a root level; *it's all about intention!* Unless your intention is pure, there will be little or no effect, so really you have to think about what it is you're after. We, as humans, have a tendency to do things only when there is a need, so if you want to move mountains with your intention, you'll need to be 100% committed to your intention and the outcome.

Age – is a state of mind, not a disease! Being conscious about what you subject your body to will allay many of the labels associated with age-related problems, but giving away your own power is worse. Perhaps age is only a problem when we give up responsibility for ourselves and take little action towards our own care?

Allergies and common intolerances –

Milk – many years ago, before hygiene regulations, pasteurisation was introduced to allay reported disease from mass-produced milk (thus destroying nutrients such as vitamins A, B6, B12, C as well as denaturing its proteins and delicate enzymes). These days, standards are stringently applied to milk-producing farmers, although it is only the farmer who can sell raw milk directly; it is illegal for supermarkets to do so. So, pasteurisation persists, but homogenisation & skimming have become the norm, thus making it very difficult for humans to obtain any goodness from milk. So let's consider how this processed milk affects humans.

Homogenization filters and presses milk fats under great pressure to create very small, uniform sized fat globules so no cream can form. This process oxidizes milk fats, reportedly making them toxic to the body. During this process, an enzyme called Xanthine Oxidase is produced which is harmful once broken down into a smaller state, and has been shown to adhere to arterial walls and be a factor in heart disease.

Because raw milk proteins are digested in the presence of milk enzymes, and the process of pasteurization and homogenization destroys or distorts these natural biological components, the human digestive tract often recognises these damaged milk proteins as antigens and may mount an immune response. This is a primary reason why processed milk is associated with mucous production (a protective mechanism by the body), leaky gut, allergies and autoimmune problems.

For those keen to redress the balance, RAW milk is available in some parts of the country *and* by post!

Ask at your local farmers market so they know there's a demand and check the web for mail order suppliers such as **www.hookandson.co.uk** and **http://www.chucklinggoat.co.uk**.

Lactose intolerance is not an allergy as it's not an immune response, but Is rather the 'norm' for any post-nursing mammal. In a large swathe of Europe, many have acquired a gene mutation that allows them to continue to produce lactose after weaning to make use of an easily available food source, but the majority of the world doesn't have this gene allele. So those who lack the ability to produce lactase, the enzyme which has the sole purpose of digesting lactose, will not be able to digest milk properly.

Milk intolerance is a different insofar as it will create varying degrees of immune response, usually from one of the many proteins in milk, or perhaps the distorted proteins in processed milk.

Wheat bread – back in the 1960's a chap stumbled across a method of bread making that could effectively generate a loaf in just under 2 hours - a significant reduction in time from the previous 4-5 hours. The industry quickly adopted this short cut to increase general production and 'keep the nation well fed'.

Some years later, it was observed that there was a sharp increase in the incidences of IBS, gluten intolerance, and other wheat-related gut problems. It seems that in the quick method, the protein from the grain is insufficiently broken down and is hard to digest. If you think this is your problem, buy bread from a traditional baker (if you can find one) or make your own using a twice-proving method. Always ensure you chew thoroughly before swallowing to ensure you mix enough saliva with the grain to aid digestion as starch digestion begins in the mouth.

Wheat contains many proteins – two main groups form the glutens, but there are others. These proteins, when split by enzymes, expose other potentially reactive substances, and coupled with the genetic variations of different cultures, it's possible to get some idea of the multiple ways that wheat can be problematic for many people. Of course, the wheat that is grown today is not the same as it was 100 years ago and has itself been honed to produce higher yields, perhaps without thought to the bioavailability of its reported nutrients, so it is up to those who consume these grains to decide if it is for them or not.

Allow yourself the space to change. Step outside of any belief systems you may have developed thus far into a zone of neutrality. Be in your own flow. As you bring in new options to try, test them out with your own intuition and see how they feel for you and if they are appropriate then make them your truth, but never be rigid in those choices. Every day is different so what you need today, may differ from yesterday or tomorrow. This is why a sharpened instinct is a useful ally.

Antibiotics There may be a time in your life when you have no choice but to succumb to the use of antibiotics,

even against your own better judgment. They may just be the short cut that your body needs to eradicate whatever stressor assails you. The good news is that there are things you can do to minimize the discomfort caused by the antibiotics that can have you feeling better in a much shorter space of time.

Slippery elm, taken about 20 minutes before your meal/ antibiotic tablet will line the gut, thus minimizing the disturbance caused by the medication; about a teaspoon mixed with water.

Marshmallow helps the stomach in a similar way, although I was told it doesn't travel to the intestine too well.

Barley water is a good gut healer and helps to alkalise the body. You can make it yourself by gently simmering ¾ cup of pearl barley with 6-8 cups of water for a few hours until you have roughly 2-3 cups of liquid. It doesn't keep well so make a fresh batch regularly.

Liquorice root is a tonic for many ailments and makes a good tea. You can buy the root ready chopped; put some into a flask & add hot water - you can keep topping up the water to extend the use of the roots. Very good for balancing blood sugar but can also be a hormone blocker. See the website

http://www.herbwisdom.com/herb-licorice-root.html for more information.

Plenty of good quality probiotics will be required immediately after the course of antibiotics in order to repopulate the gut with 'good' bacteria and return the flora to a balanced state; failure to do so will lead to the candida in your body going on the rampage. **Saccharomyces boulardii** is a yeast that can be useful both during and after the antibiotics as it's not destroyed by the them.

One more thing, whilst suffering with any type of infection, and until you're fully recovered, it's wise to stay off all foods with added sugar (i.e. unnatural); sugars (and alcohol) feed bacteria, yeasts and viruses, thus slowing down recovery.

Attitude – we view the world around us through the filters of our belief systems and conditioning, but it is our attitude that largely decides how we choose to respond to it. Although our mood can sometimes be affected by our internal chemistry, we can generally choose how we enter into each day. Do we moan about anything and everything, or do we accept what the river of life brings our way? One thing humans are gifted with is free will...

Autogenic Training

Autogenic (self-generated) training is a self-help relaxation technique developed by J H Schulz, a German psychiatrist, back in 1932 in order to allay many stress-induced disorders. It was subsequently popularised in North America by Wolfgang Luthe who worked with Schulz to further develop the training. After further investigation, Luthe developed a method of autogenic abreaction, allowing for previously repressed emotions to be released.

The main precept is that Autogenics is a safe and simple technique for use by the individual as a vehicle to reduce or manage stress-related issues such as anxiety, mild depression, fatigue, sleep problems, IBS, chronic pain and asthma. The training involves the repetition of key phrases to relax independent parts of the body in sequence. Each session lasts for 15 minutes and is performed 2 or 3 times a day in order to encourage a release from any manifestation of stress. Autogenic Training aims to engage mind and body in reversing the stress response, which in turn allows for the inherent health-balancing mechanisms within the body to respond naturally.

To begin, sit or lie comfortably where you will not be disturbed, close your eyes and begin to observe your breath. Observe the way your body moves with each breath and begin the process of letting go, mentally following the exhale, rest in the pause between each breath, then allow the inhale to begin itself.

Follow – rest – allow, follow – rest – allow, all the while extending each breath without effort. Now take each of the phrases below and repeat them silently three times to yourself:

"My right hand and arm are heavy and warm."

"My left hand and arm are heavy and warm."

"Both my hands and arms are heavy and warm."

"I am calm and relaxed."

Now move your attention into the right foot and leg;

"My right foot and leg are heavy and warm."

"My left foot and leg are heavy and warm."

"Both my feet and legs are heavy and warm"

"I am calm and relaxed."

Continue to observe the breath, allowing the body to relax further, and say to yourself "My breath breathes me".

"The muscles of my neck and jaw are soft and supple."

"My lower back is warm, relaxed and comfortable."

"My entire body is calm and at ease."

"My mind is quiet and serene."

"My forehead is cool."

"Knowing how to relax, I move through my day with ease."

Now count back from 3 to 1 as you return your awareness to the room, before seeing yourself moving through your day with peace and ease.

The above is a self-help version of the autogenic training that is taught through a trained therapist, but is a good way to begin, and for some may be all they need.

The British Autogenic Society – **www.autogenic-therapy.org.uk** - provides a list of trained therapists who teach this tool. Alternatively, there are several books available upon the subject and videos on YouTube for anyone wishing to teach themselves.

B

Balance – seek mental, emotional and physical balance in whatever ways suit you. Whatever your form of work, notice how common it is in today's society to bow to the pressures of what we *should* be doing, even if we work for ourselves. Whatever we do, we need to include other activities that stimulate the parts of us that we're not using regularly. So, if you're nailed to a computer most of the day, some form of exercise and walking are essential in order to release some endorphins and balance the emotions. When we fail to keep this balance, we can become stressed and depressed, losing perspective. Basically, there needs to be movement in all areas of our life, at all times, or we stagnate. Again, I recommend you tune in to your intuition to guide you.

Bathing – hugely underestimated for its usefulness as a health aid, and a great place to perform a weekly maintenance session. A standard size bath is a great place to work on your skin with a flannel - toning, exfoliating and performing general maintenance. A sitz bath, for the lower half of the body, can be both soothing and therapeutic, warm or cold, and helps those conditions such as constipation, haemorrhoids, anal fissures, and post rectal surgery. The benefit of using a sitz bath is that the temperature of the water can be easily controlled, or even alternated, whilst avoiding the light-headed effect that may occur in a full sized bath.

Beauty – humans are the only species of the animal kingdom able to behold beauty. You can use this to consciously uplift yourself by looking at something that *you* find truly beautiful. Breathe in that feeling of upliftment, allowing it to fill you up so you can take it away with you into your daily life. It's not just a momentary thing, if you take beauty into your heart, positive chemical changes can and do occur.

Biorhythms – an interesting tool to gauge your mental, physical and emotional cycles. The system originally came about in the late 19th century, upon observations of a *physical* cycle of 23 days, an *emotional* cycle of 28 days and later, an *intellectual* cycle of 33 days. It is possible to mathematically calculate your current position using the above numbers in each cycle, counting from the day you were born, giving the current positive or negative energetic value. In the 1970's, this system gained popularity and early computational systems were devised to automate the calculating process. Now, free online versions are available for you to try. Maybe give it a try for 6 months to see whether you can feel the energetic swing from the positive to the negative, and how this information might be useful to you in your daily life. I currently use

http://www.biorhythmonline.com/?lang=en-gb but other sites are of course available.

Boundaries – Decide where your boundaries lie; make them clear and build on them as your foundation. They will need periodic amendment throughout life but they will provide a guideline of how you live and the kind of attention you attract into your life. Value yourself and don't be made to feel guilty because you've had the courage to communicate decisions that are right for *you*. If you feel your boundaries have been violated, you may experience a very natural surge of anger as this emotion is used to reinstate your boundaries.

Breathing – adequate oxygen in the body is necessary to achieve a balanced environment for your cells. Lack of oxygen from inefficient breathing makes the body's environment more acidic. If the blood becomes very acidic, the respiratory centre in the medulla oblongata will be affected, resulting in a further decrease in breathing – catch 22. Use bodywork, exercise, breath work and regular stretching to maintain the movement that supports the action of the diaphragm. The wall of the abdomen works antagonistically with the diaphragm during breathing. If your abdomen doesn't move in and out as you breathe, you're not using all of your lungs. Deep breathing means that if you rest your hands on your abdomen with fingertips touching, inhaling will move your fingertips apart. A good exercise at bedtime is to do 9 cycles of breathing - in to the count of 8, hold for 2 seconds, then breathe out for a count of 8, hold for 2 seconds – chances are you'll be asleep before you've finished. Deep breathing decreases stress naturally.

C

Candida – inhabits the intestinal tract of us all in but can become overgrown and pathogenic when a person's body is out of balance. When Candida changes to its pathogenic, mycelial form its roots can permeate the gut lining, causing leaky gut syndrome and releasing acidic mycotoxins into the person's body. Many things in modern society can throw the body off-balance. Some of those things include: antibiotics, vaccines, stress, toxins in our food and environment, birth control pills and other medications, not to mention the effects of a highly refined, sugar-rich diet or long term alcohol consumption. Hormonal shifts such as pregnancy and menopause can also be precipitators of imbalance, encouraging Candida overgrowth.

In my experience, another common condition, **hypochlorhydria** (low production of gastric acid in the stomach), can also lead to an overgrowth of candida because it feeds off food that has not been broken down effectively in the gut, even if the diet does not contain high amounts of sugars. Imagine this going on for years... It is worth considering supplementing a good HCl if restricting key foods/nutrients has failed to have much effect, or you've noticed other symptoms associated with hypochlorhydria (such as reflux).

It's a good idea to do some research on anti-inflammatory, sugar control and dysbiosis diets. These healing diets have much in common with a candida diet and may work well for your system. Remember, the key to clearing candida is to heal your digestive system, kill the candida using caprylic acid and herbs, avoid foods that feed the candida, and support your liver in clearing the toxins that result from the die-off.

These days, there is much written on the subject of candida overgrowth, so do please do your own research if you think you have this problem. Simply cutting out all sugars and sugar producing foods/drinks for 2 weeks will enable you to feel a difference i.e. caffeine raises blood sugar so feeds candida.

Chi machine was created in Japan by Keiichi Ohashi in 1988. The original concept for the machine was taken from the Aikido 'goldfish exercise' – an oscillating fishtail movement that stimulates the lymphatic system and is thought to introduce more oxygen into the body. Research done at Flinders University in Adelaide in 2000 showed a reduction in pain and swelling, plus some weight loss during clinical trials focusing on secondary lymphedema when using this machine.

The Chi machine is used whilst lying flat on the floor and can be built up from just a few minutes to 15 minutes at a time. I can report that following a 10 minute session, the lymphatic system is literally buzzing and a great feeling of relaxation descends upon the whole body (usually followed by a few zzz's). As long as there are no serious knee issues (the side to side movement could agitate a problematic joint) I believe this machine would benefit any who favour a more passive approach to stimulating their lymphatic system.

The fluids within the human body form a transportation system for whatever needs to move around the body as well as the means by which toxins are removed. Therefore the body *must* have movement in order to stay healthy, hence why the fishtail movement is so beneficial. Conditions whereby the fluids of the body are allowed to stagnate for any length of time pave the way for a diseased state.

I mention the Chi machine here because not only can it be used to improve the healing of conditions or injuries where an increase in circulation is beneficial, but I have found that it clearly helps to improve the *stuck* energy situation that can arise during day to day living from things like a build up of tension, a lack of exercise, too much time 'in the head' and the effects of inadequate personal boundaries.

Cholesterol – "this myth began a couple of decades ago when researchers found that those dying from heart disease frequently had elevated blood cholesterol levels, as well as fatty plaque, called atheromas, which clog up the arteries of the heart muscle. These atheromas consisted of prolific smooth muscle cells filled with, and surrounded by, fatty sludge containing high levels of cholesterol.

Medical authorities believed that cutting down on our cholesterol intake would lower blood cholesterol levels and therefore reduce the risk of heart disease. However biochemists were sceptical of this idea, after all, the liver produces most of our cholesterol requirements and only about 1.5% comes from the intake/breakdown of our food, the excess being excreted in the bile.

Despite what we've been led to believe, cholesterol is a very valuable substance, providing the basis for the synthesis of steroid hormones and vitamin D, and is a major component of cells in the brain and nervous systems. However, deficiencies of the emulsifier lecithin or sulphur amino acids may create an accumulation of cholesterol as gallstones.

So you can see that it is very important for us to have enough cholesterol. Furthermore, "some wasting diseases such as cancer, are associated with cholesterol deficiency, and hypoglycaemias are commonly found to have low cholesterol levels."

The above excerpt is taken from the site of Walter Last at http://www.health-science-spirit.com/ where you can read much more about this and other health related matters.

Circadian rhythms – a built-in cycle affecting most living things over a day, a season or a year. These processes are endogenous; they adapt to external stimuli, the most common being daylight. However, the modern day extended usage of light-emitting computer/gadget screens used way beyond the normal hours of daylight are responsible for at least some disruption of sleep in humans. Circadian rhythms affect digestive and elimination processes, as well as hormonal release and can be disturbed by stress.

The diagram below gives some idea of how we can be affected:

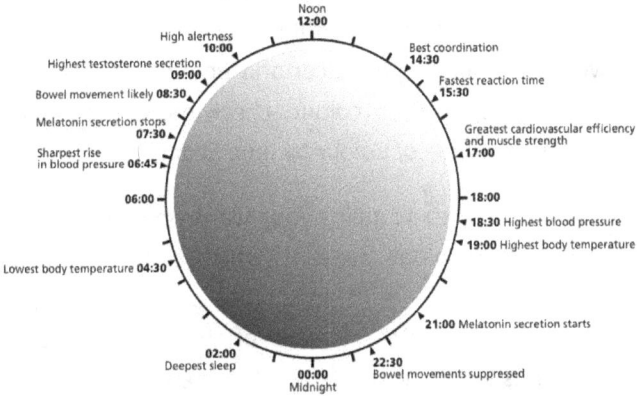

Coconut oil – is one of the finest fats to eat. It does not go rancid at room temperature and speeds up cellular metabolism. It can be used in cooking, added to smoothies or as a spread instead of butter. More recently, coconut oil is being lauded as a treatment for Alzheimers disease. There are many on the market but not all taste nice. My favourite is from http://coconoil.co.uk/

Colour – an important part of everyday life. Imagine if the world were only seen in monochrome; the lack of differentiation, with nothing for the eyes to gain upliftment from would make for a bland world indeed.

Colour is therapeutic, each shade carrying its own vibration, and can be used to support your personality and mood. It is a powerful healer in its own right, as well as a useful re-balancer and energizer. If you are drawn to work with colour, check out the book *The Secret Language of Colour* by Inna Segal.

It is a good idea to tailor your wardrobe over time to reflect your colour 'season' (which colours best suit your skin tone). Cull unsuitable colours from your wardrobe and bring in more of the ones that uplift you, thus enabling you to work more readily with the colours that complement you on a daily basis. I arrange my clothes into colour bands in the wardrobe, allowing for easy selection at the beginning of the day; I find it hard to plan what to wear ahead of time as I have to 'feel' what colour I am upon waking.

Constipation – usually has a few causes – insufficient water intake or incorrect diet i.e. heavy in dry and fatty foods and lacking the protein needed to stimulate peristalsis, plus a lack of routine.
I suffered from this condition whilst working shifts. In order to get things moving, my herbalist prescribed the use of a herbal blend containing cascara sagrada. Whilst that guaranteed the release of waste from my body for some years, it was only when I reverted to an omnivorous diet that I found normal peristalsis returned.

D

Dance – Is about moving your body to any music that makes you feel good, even if you've got two left feet. Music has the ability to rouse the soul and lift the heart, and cannot fail to bring joy and excitement to living. Dancing has been recognised by BUPA to be "socially inclusive and known to maintain both the physical and mental health of all who participate".

Deodorant –Sweating is a natural function that cools the skin and carries waste from the body, so it is unwise to suppress it more than occasionally. When we sweat, the bacteria on the skin breaks down the acids in the sweat, producing the odour we associate with profuse sweating. The many anti-perspirants sold today block the pores of the skin and increase the body's toxic load. However, the aluminium-free deodorants help to prevent odour whilst allowing perspiration, although a pinch of bicarbonate of soda would do the same for just a few pence.

Detoxing – both mentally and physically is an essential part of life. As our eating, living and social habits change, we move away from this very natural process. If we choose to eat refined/modified foods as opposed to whole natural foods, it follows that we have to work harder to preserve our internal balance. Therefore the 'you are what you eat' model encourages us to consider the effects of what we consume. Of course, we must also consider what we absorb *energetically*, the effects of which are just as important. Just as you tidy your home, so you should tidy your inner world.

Diaphragm – an important muscle for breathing that is affected by posture and emotions. At the front, it is attached to the sternum and lower ribs and at the rear it attaches via a flat ligament to the lumbar spine. The action of the diaphragm during deep breathing or yoga helps massage our internal organs and keep things moving. Bad posture, injury or illness, where an upright posture is no longer maintained, has the effect of limiting inspiration and the body quickly changes to a more acidic medium (this once happened to me within an hour, following a fall that pulled some spinal ligaments).

Digestion – is all about taking in, processing and absorbing that which nourishes us, in order that our body can perform the many functions that make us healthy. A shortfall in any part of this chain will undermine long term health.

- **Chewing** – breaks down and increases the surface area of ingested food, thus enabling HCl (stomach acid) and enzymes to work effectively. Failing to chew your food adequately can lead to **indigestion** (stomach), **bloating** (fermentation in the gut, producing excess gas and causing discomfort) and poor availability of nutrients. Taking more time to eat has advantages.

- **HCl** – stomach acidity needs to be enough to break down the macronutrients – carbohydrate, protein, fats. If stomach pH is too high (i.e. too alkaline, caused by stress/increasing age), this does not happen effectively, and the barrier against bacterium, viruses etc. is weak and bacterial/fungal overgrowth that can occur, producing excess gas in the small intestine. This increases abdominal pressure, causing distension and problems like reflux/heartburn. Weak stomach acid can give rise to chronic bowel issues like IBS, tiredness, food intolerances, etc. and may have been going on for many years. You can read about how antacids actually worsen this problem on http://chriskresser.com/how-your-antacid-drug-is-making-you-sick-part-b and further information about the digestive process on http://www.ion.ac.uk/information/onarchives/improvedigestion

If you've tried waiting until you have real hunger pangs before eating and you still have weak digestion, you could try supplementing **betaine HCl & Pepsin** (the main constituent of gastric acid). Experiment with the amount you take, depending upon the density/size of the meal to be consumed. Notice any changes 1-2 hours after eating and general improvements within a week.

103

- **Absorption** – gut health needs to be maintained in order to absorb the nutrients in the food we've eaten (assuming it's been broken down effectively). If the bowel walls are silted up, the ability of the body to obtain the nutrients it needs are diminished, and the tendency is to pull toxins into the blood stream (one cause of headaches) from impacted fecal matter. As a result of shift work, I came to rely upon a herbal formula containing **cascara sagrada** to regulate the passage of matter through the bowel, but I also massaged my abdomen regularly in order to aid this process and help to release tension. Occasional colonic irrigation can be helpful in correcting and healing the gut, as can home enemas. NB: I found psyllium husks and seeds to be irritants to my gut - a good reminder to test any advice out for myself.
- See also **Enzymes** and **Gut Health** below.

Distractions - all the many things we fill our lives with that divert us from what contributes to it.

Dowsing – see the chapter **My Toolbox** for more information.

Dreams – lucid or otherwise, often contain messages that are helpful in understanding yourself and what you're going through. The interpretation of dreams is often symbolic and pertinent only to you and how you see the world. Keep a notebook by the bed and write down 7 words as you wake at the end of the dream, then flesh out later in order to decipher the meaning.

E

Eating, thoughts on –

* *"If you eat what's good for you, there's not much room for what you fancy"* – old saying from Granny.

* Eat only as much as *your* body can actually use at that time – anything else turns to fat.

* Make (*almost*) everything that passes your lips count.

* A small amount of good quality food beats any amount of junk food.

* Junk food is a filler with no nutritional value; ask *Why* before you buy.

* A diet can be observed in action by watching how your body and emotions respond a few hours later.

* Regular mealtimes, with sufficient time between to fully burn what you ate previously are more likely to lead to balance.

* Eating 'proper' meals reduces the need for snacking.

Eating seasonal, locally grown foods is the ideal to aim for – the site below gives a Chinese perspective on this, along with some interesting effects:
http://www.shen-nong.com/eng/lifestyles/food_diet_advice_season.html

Electro-magnetic pollution – devices such as computers and TV's are always on 'standby' even when not switched on, and still emit electro-magnetic pollution. All electrical devices around the home should be unplugged when not in use so as to avoid the continual build-up of this type of energy which ultimately depletes the natural energy field of humans. Having your bed against an adjoining neighbours wall can also be a factor as you may be picking up their EMF's.

Emotions – "Emotional energy works at a higher speed than thought. This is because the feeling world operates at a higher rate than the mind. We evaluate everything as we perceive it; we think about it afterwards.

If emotional energy works faster than the mind, how can we expect to manage our emotions with our thoughts? It takes more than the mind to manage emotions – the heart's coherent energy is required as well.

Heart coherence helps balance our emotional state – it aligns head and heart to facilitate higher brain function, which appears to create a direct link to intuition. Intuition bypasses mental analysis and gives us direct perception, independent of any reasoning process. Intuition gives us clarity on how to direct and manage our feelings before we invest emotional energy in them.

One of the main purposes of emotion in the human system is to provide a means of expression for core heart feelings. But since "heart intelligence isn't developed in most people, the mind more often hijacks our emotional energy and uses it to express *its* perceptions and reactions". *From the book The HeartMath Solution by Doc Childre & Howard Martin.*

Emotions are not something we need to deny or suppress. They are ever-present in our lives, and can affect our health and lives when left unchecked. As someone who likes to delve deeply into every experience that gets my attention, I realise that like Alice falling down the rabbit hole, there is a fine line between following where an emotion takes me, and over-indulging in its melodrama to the extent where rationale is hard to return to.

Approximately half of the population live their lives through an emotional filter whilst the rest may struggle to understand their own reflected emotional states. Neither is wrong, yet many struggle to comprehend each others' differences in the emotional field.

Emotions add colour, texture and joy to our very existence, and life would be bland without them. We need emotions, just as we need an ego.

A useful tool for balancing the emotions is the range of Bach Flower remedies – we discover which of the range works for us and keep a few in for when we need rebalancing.

Enema – a very fine tool that was well used by the medical profession until it fell out of favour. When waste material travels too slowly through the intestines or you become constipated, putrefaction occurs; this material can cling to the bowel wall over time, creating longer term issues. Constipation is damaging to every cell and organ of the body, not just the intestines. Our bodies are designed to absorb whatever is in the digestive tract... good or bad. An enema is used to flush out the colon, which is a good idea when you consider that the average person carries many pounds of non-eliminated waste in the large intestine.

An enema cleans up the colon and induces bowel movements, leaving you feeling healthier and clear-headed *immediately*. See the Revital website at https://www.revital.co.uk/Enema_Kit

I have found that a daily warm water enema (for 10 days), from the first sign of a problem, can be used to tackle some bowel problems in their early stages, as it provides a clean environment for the required healing to take place naturally. It is certainly more preferable to taking medicinal products that invariably disrupt the sensitive natural mechanisms.

Enzymes – Enzymes are proteins that facilitate key metabolic actions in the body. These actions are essential in fuelling all systems of the body; all of your cells, organs, bones, muscles, and tissues are run by enzymes. Therefore your energy levels, your ability to utilize vitamins and minerals, your immune system are all facilitated by these enzymes.

Some enzymes are produced in the body whilst others are taken in raw food. The body cannot make all enzymes, therefore we need to include them in our diet. Unfortunately, processing and cooking destroys enzymes found in food. A diet consisting *entirely* of cooked food places a lot of stress on the pancreas and other endocrine glands of the body. If the digestion that takes place before food reaches the small intestine is minimal i.e. with low stomach acid, food lacking in enzymes, or inefficient chewing - more stress is placed on the endocrine systems and the process of digestion is weakened.

The digestive system and general health can be aided by supplementing *good* digestive enzymes (not all enzymes are equal – check the strength against the price, and experiment with how many you need to take to achieve the desired effect – a good enzyme formulation usually requires 1-2 per meal).

It is common these days for enzyme production in the

body and via food intake to be low, so supplementing can help to ensure better energy and long-term health as your absorption inevitably improves.

Essential Oils – are the liquid aromatic extractions sourced from plants, flowers, trees, roots, fruits and grasses. The extraction methods are devised to carefully preserve the potent plant properties and produce a concentrated liquid. The more sensitive the extraction method, the more expensive the oil, rose petals being a prime example in the 'absolute' form. The most common form of extraction, steam distillation, is too harsh for rose petals, so they require the more gentle use of CO_2 (carbon dioxide) in order to retain the light *and* heavy molecules that give the full spectrum of the aroma.

Essential oils are not simply used for their medicinal properties, of which there are many; the food and cosmetics industry has employed them for hundreds of years, although in recent decades, many of these have been phased out in favour of cheaper synthetic 'flavours'.

A true plant essence has the ability to involve the user in its own synergistic qualities, drawing you deep into its innate wisdom with confidence. All we the users have to do is allow our own instinct to direct us to the correct match for our needs. The power of a good essential oil is without question something that many of us can resonate with to balance mood, restore harmony, to calm and nurture. All are within the ability of these wonderful gifts from nature. If you decide to place your trust in essential oils, allowing your instinct to join the guiding hand of nature, you will be surprised and delighted by how neatly they fit into your life, providing the most suitable answer to your problems, be they mental, emotional or physical, just when your mind had run out of answers.

The wisdom of good essential oils (there are some who produce liquids that do little to reflect the plant kingdoms' power) cannot be denied. The skill of the individual and the aromatherapist lies in matching the vibration of the oil to the vibration of the client/user in order to restore balance. I refer not only to physical issues here, for it is well known that they have the power to balance emotions also. There have been times when I have received a smell psychically to help me overcome a particular situation – cinnamon to ease high emotion, vanilla for grief, eucalyptus for anger - all to great effect.

When you wish to build your own store of essential oils, allow yourself to be guided by what *you* are drawn to rather than what is written, for the qualities in those oils will be called by your own innate needs. Store them in a cool place or even the refrigerator; good quality oils can keep for some years, but some are so volatile their qualities keep for a much shorter time. Take one or two key oils with you when you travel, for they are adaptable to all situations where a helping hand is required and you will derive great comfort from knowing you have them, like a trusted friend always beside you. If I were to recommend two oils, it would be lavender and tea tree, simply for availability.

Exercise – can be anything you enjoy that gets your body moving. 'Use it or lose it' certainly applies to muscle tone and range of movement, but it doesn't have to be excessive or onerous. Cleaning the house is exercise, as is gardening or washing the car. Any exercise that gets you out of breath and increases your oxygen uptake will therefore contribute to making you less acidic. Frequency is the key; aim for 3 times per week and supplement with regular 30-minute walks, daily if possible, but whatever the case, do try to make it enjoyable.

F

Fats – my training has taught me that the best fats to consume for good health are ghee (clarified butter), coconut oil and good quality olive oil, as well as the saturated fats in (good quality) flesh foods. Mary Enig and Sally Fallon have done much to correct the huge amount of misinformation about fats that has been bandied around for the past few decades by putting out good research - see their books 'Nourishing

Traditions' and 'Eat Fat, Lose Fat' for more information. Make friends with fat and learn what works for you. For instance, coconut oil (my favourite is Coconoil) increases cellular metabolism, so can actually help you to lose weight, not to mention it's many other benefits. See the piece above on Cholesterol.

Fermented foods – a method of food preparation used before refrigeration, which increases the nutrient value of foods - Sauerkraut being one of the most obvious. Recipe suggestions and information on fermentation can be found in 'Rawsome' by Brigitte Mars and 'Nourishing Traditions' by Sally Fallon, plus many other internet sites.

Fever – is a useful house-cleaning tool for the body. Fever is seen less and less these days as people are used to self-medicating, but may still be seen among the offspring of the informed and courageous.

The body requires a certain amount of energy to create a fever and so it is no surprise that previously healthy individuals may occasionally be struck down by something as simple as the common cold, which then turns into something of more *apparent* seriousness. Because people these days aren't used to allowing a disease process to run its course, they panic and take a suppressant instead of allowing the fever to do what it was meant to. Allowing the body to heat up to a relatively high temperature for a short time effectively kills off any bacterium, viruses or bugs within the body, including some that may have been hanging around for quite some time. In general, much better health can be seen *after* this uninterrupted process is complete.

Following a fever, eat carefully for the next day or two while the clean-up process is finished, and drink enough water. There's probably a good reason why this situation occurred in the bigger scheme of things, so enjoy doing nothing except observing the wonder of nature as your body corrects itself.

Flexibility – if we work at being flexible in the mind, it is more likely we can be flexible in the body. Similarly, painful joints can indicate a resistance to moving forward in life (read also about the effects of fluoride below).

Fluoride – a known toxin that is wantonly added to our water and toothpaste. Ionic fluoride is not the same as organic <u>fluorine</u>; the latter *contributes* to teeth and bone health. Ionic fluoride <u>is toxic</u> in very small doses (see the warning on the side of toothpaste tubes re swallowing the stuff). Some scientists noticed that organic fluorine is required with calcium and molybdenum for healthy teeth and bones so extrapolating this, decided more fluorine 'could' mean healthier teeth (not proven). Hence they suggested adding *fluoride* to the water supplies, even though the health effects are <u>not</u> the same as with organic fluorine.

Ionic fluoride does not contribute to the formation of teeth and bones and instead causes the over stimulation of the parathyroid glands, resulting in abnormal bone growth, calcification of tendons and ligaments and interrupts the process which generates energy in cells, probably because it reduces iodine in the body. (Fluoride is a by-product of paper and aluminium manufacturing and is expensive to dispose of. Draw your own conclusions.)

Food choices – prolific availability of previously uncommon foods, coupled with media exposure about their so-called benefits, has meant that some folks fall into the trap of over-consuming foods they *believe* to be health giving. This practice does not encourage balance and is contrary to the natural cycle of availability. Is what you are eating normally available in this country/at this time, and are you genetically predisposed to do well on this food? Be guided by your instinct rather than the media, and remember – moderation in all things.

Free will – something we all have access to. It is the device that shapes our past, present and future and works best with mindful application.

Friends – worth investing in. Some come and go, whilst others will be with you for life, but there's no doubt that they are the greatest asset a person can have, and life is richer because of them.

G

Gall bladder – a small sac below the liver that collects bile in order to concentrate it. Bile is necessary to emulsify the fats in our food so we can absorb them. Modern grazing habits and popular diets mean that frequently the gall bladder is not emptied effectively as food passes through the duodenum, so what is left behind becomes stagnant.

Once or twice a year, a simple pectin-based cleanse can be employed to soften the stones, enabling them to be 'flushed' painlessly from the body. If you've never done this kind of thing before, the guidance of a practitioner might be helpful, at least for the first time. If more people were aware of this procedure, perhaps the need for the removal of many gall bladders could be averted. The ever-wise Google has many suggestions for a "liver & gallbladder flush".

Garlic – nature's finest antibiotic, antimicrobial, cleanser and purifier. If you're feeling under the weather and feel the need for strong medicine, my experience is that there's nothing better than raw garlic. 1-3 cloves, finely chopped and added to a little water first thing in the morning, just before your breakfast will work wonders. The main active ingredient – allicin – remains active in the body for up to 60 hours, so you don't have to take it every day to benefit from its actions. I have found that it can negate anything else you're taking at the same time though, so be aware if you're on essential medication.

Genetics – browse around your family tree, checking out any obvious health problems. See how these could translate into any problems you may have and whether these may be learned (i.e. copied behaviour) or genetic predispositions. I would suggest to you that nothing is fixed; your gene expression is directly affected by your own choices and attitude to life.

Geopathic stress – refers to the study of earth energies and their effect upon human health. Although some energies are believed to be beneficial, others are detrimental. Basically, various underground formations, such as subterranean water currents, specific mineral deposits, or different fault lines emit specific electromagnetic fields that can be harmful for a human dwelling. If you are just passing through an area with geopathic stress, there will be little or no concern. However if your house and especially your bed is positioned over earth grid lines, it is likely you will experience a steady decline in health and/or energy, the ability to sleep well or the emergence of conditions that you previously didn't have. Many cases of cancer have been reported where geopathic stress was thought to be the reason.

Corrective action can be taken by placing copper at the points where the grid lines enter your property, but the best solution is to either move beds/favourite chairs away from grid lines or, if that's not possible, look into ways of moving house. Good health cannot be achieved whilst the body is experiencing this kind of stressor. You can read more on this website; http://www.spaceclearing.com/web/html/links/geopa thic-stress.html

Gravity – as an ever-present force, there will inevitably be an effect on the body. As we age and our own life force decreases, the effect of gravity increases. Explore ways you can reverse the effects of gravity upon your body, especially in the legs. Be inventive - you don't have to own an inversion table, but neither should you give in and do nothing. One of the best ways I know to stimulate the circulation in your legs (and body) is to give yourself a good rub down with a flannel during your bath/shower.

Growing your own – now is the time to experiment – anywhere you have some soil, you can grow something. Try a couple of vegetable items you enjoy, even if its cherry tomatoes or chillies in a window box – have a go.

Guru – be your own - turn inwards to where your personal guru awaits.

Gut health – imperative for clear thinking and a sense of well-being. Gut health can always be improved by clearing old emotional issues, regular breathing exercises and being more relaxed. The latter may need lots of practice as layers of tension may have been building for years. Massaging your own abdomen helps but so does eating correctly. Tending to your digestive requirements and using digestive supplements when the time comes to give your body a helping hand is recommended. If you regularly have gurgling or discomfort in your abdomen, you're not going to feel settled or peaceful; rather you'll always have an undercurrent of anxiety running in the background.

H

Habit – the human brain naturally seeks patterns and enjoys following familiarity. When an action is performed more than once, a habit is in the making. This principle works just as well to create good habits or over-write unhelpful ones – it simply involves being mindful of each step as you move or act in a different way.

Headaches – are frequently a sign of blood-borne toxicity, be it from over-indulgence, dehydration or infection, so it's wise to take action instead of a painkiller.

1. Drink a glass of water.

2. If the headache is due to a toxic rush from over-indulgence in rich food/alcohol or even detoxing, try the following:

   • the homeopathic remedy **Nux.Vom.**

   • the amino acid **L-Ornithine** is superb for cleaning the blood of partially digested proteins, something that is necessary if the liver is overloaded and the blood is carrying too much large particulate.

   • **Plant-based antioxidants** are helpful during a detox, whether it be intentional or accidental (going too long without food).

   • If you know the headache is due to chemical overload, **activated Charcoal** is really good at 'mopping up'. I take 2-3 capsules at once.

3. If a virus is suspected (first signs: unusual ache at the base of the neck and/or sacrum), try applying some neat essential oil (**lavender or ravensara**) to

the back of the neck and base of the spine; you should feel an improvement within 20 minutes.

4. Best but least favoured solution – a mild coffee enema to free up the liver energy - it does wonders to clear both gut and head.

If it's a 'stress' headache that's created by muscular tension, remove yourself from the stressor and employ a relaxation technique.

Healing – achieved on many levels and in many ways. It could be something as simple as talking to someone who makes you feel calm, or it could be one of the energetic modalities available with someone you've put your trust in. The effect is to rebalance your physical and energetic bodies, which in turn restores health. Healing can be used to combat painful situations or to avert them. Go to where you are drawn, trusting your intuition to guide you.

Hemi-sync - *Hemi-Sync* is short for *Hemispheric Synchronization,* also known as brainwave synchronization. The founder, Robert Monroe, indicated that using audio patterns containing binaural beats, the two hemispheres of the brain could be synchronized to evoke certain effects. Hemi-Sync has been used for many purposes, including relaxation and sleep induction, learning and memory aids, helping those with physical and mental difficulties, and reaching altered states of consciousness through the use of sound.

Human Design – Human Design uses your birth data to calculate a rave chart, also known as your Bodygraph. This is based on the science of Neutrinos, tiny particles that carry mass and information which determine your unique imprinting. The Human Design System is a synthesis of two streams of science, traditional and modern. The traditional sciences: Astrology, the Chakra system, the Kabbalah and the I'Ching, are the traditional elements in the synthesis that is Human Design.

Combined with the modern science of reading the genetic code, Human Design offers you a profound insight into how you are designed to navigate the material world. In my humble opinion, this is a very useful tool when working out you and yours, as taking the 'givens' out of the puzzle leaves fewer questions, and helps provide understanding about family and personal interactions.

Humility – along with Acceptance, are two attributes we would all do well to cultivate if we are to live the happy and contented life that we seek.

I

Incontinence – can be influenced by the Autonomic Nervous System, in much the same way as reflux from the stomach, where the valves of both are dominated by the Sympathetic half of the ANS. The ANS can be strengthened and balanced by correct nutrition and long-term reduction of stress.

Indigestion and IBS – see **digestion** above.

Insecticides – many crops are sprayed heavily during their production but lettuce, strawberries and grapes are among the worst. If you learn to dowse, you can measure how much of an effect this factor has on your particular system and which to avoid. Failing that, it is best to go organic.

Instinct – probably the most valuable asset you'll ever possess; it's the small, quiet voice within that will speak on a matter only once and if you're not listening, you can miss it. Instinct communicates with the heart to process incoming information, and gives you the only guidance you can rely on. Practice using your instinct every day until your 'gut' feeling becomes automatic; simply by looking at something, you know whether it's good or bad for you.

Iodine
"Medical textbooks contain several vital pieces of misinformation about the essential element Iodine, which may have caused more human misery and death than both world wars combined." Dr. Guy Abraham

"Every 17 minutes, every drop of blood in our body flushes through our thyroid, and if our thyroid has an

adequate supply of iodine, blood-borne bacteria and viruses are killed off as the blood passes through the thyroid." Walter Last.

When I read something like the above two comments, I immediately want to know more, especially anything from the pen of Walter Last. I have mentioned it here because I suspect many people rarely think of using iodine for health, except for wound cleaning or water purification. So let's look at a few of the benefits and functions of iodine.

The benefits of iodine in the body are significant, yet it is the least understood of all the essential trace elements. Having sufficient iodine in the body means you can;

- Maintain a good energy level all day
- Maintain normal weight
- Live without aches and pains
- Maintain a positive and uplifted attitude
- Have a clear memory
- Are able to tolerate cold
- Have normal bowel movements
- Have restful sleep
- Have normal skin and nails.

Iodine is not only needed for a healthy thyroid, but also by the breasts, ovaries and prostate gland. Women who are deficient in iodine are more prone to breast and thyroid cancer, but iodine also has a key role in protecting the body from such poisons as fluoride and bromide. Iodine aids elimination of metals like lead and mercury from the body, and has a supportive effect on antioxidant and immune activity.

Iodine is deadly for single cell microorganisms, killing them with a simple chemical reaction and is a potent germicide with low toxicity to tissues, so it could be said that it is more valuable than antibiotics.

My own use of Lugol's Iodine has been to take 1-2 drops in water in the morning. The more deficient I was, the more noticeable the effect, especially how uplifted I felt. I now take it once or twice a week.

http://www.iodine-resource.com is a very helpful site about all things on and around iodine by Jill Van Eps of Florida, following her own journey through iodine deficiency. It is certainly worth a read.

L

Learning lessons – they come at you thick and fast in early life, usually decreasing in frequency as we wise up and learn to duck when we see one on the horizon. Everything we find difficult in life can be seen as a lesson, a gift or a learning opportunity, so grasp the nettle and get on with it before the opportunity to learn has vanished. You'll be wiser and stronger once you see the point of the lesson.

Love – the utopia we all strive to discover in this life, usually outside of ourselves. It can take many years to finally arrive at the realization that as our birthright, it was always right there inside of us, just waiting...

Lymphatic system – is a filtration system that carries proteins and waste in plasma from between the cells, cleaning the fluid as it passes through lymph nodes, before returning it to the vascular system. The lymph system also plays a major role in immunity.

Symptoms of sluggish lymphatic system include persistent dull inner pelvic and backache, neck and/or shoulder aching, abdominal distension, and aching joints in the morning, plus changes to vision. Oedema, especially of the extremities, occurs later.

The 'aching' mentioned above, is a result of the increased pressure to nerve endings, which is why aching is often more pronounced in the morning after a poor night's sleep, usually felt in the shoulders and neck, sometimes with a dull headache. A late, fat-laden evening meal puts a lot of stress on the lymphatic system at a time when the energy of the body to process this load is reduced – hence can be the cause of snoring or sleep apnoea. Anyone who suffers from these problems should work on strengthening their lymphatic system, i.e. drinking regular infusions of **cleavers**. If you wish to gather your own cleavers, gather them around May time, before they flower and away from the roadsides or animals. Dry your gathered cleavers thoroughly and then roughly chop them before storing in jars or bags.

One of the best ways to stimulate your lymphatic system is to make daily use of a rebounder (small, firm trampoline). Another useful gadget is the 'chi' machine; you lay down with ankles placed on the machine, which then oscillates from side to side, sending a fish tail movement through the body; (see more information above on the Chi machine). Regular exercise is certainly a must to keep lymph moving as we age, as is the reduction of the nutritional load down to only what your body can easily use each day.

M

Macronutrients – the 3 macronutrients that form the basis for our diet are protein, fat, and carbohydrate. Each meal and snack should contain an element from all these groups. The source of these three groups would ideally be as close to their original form as possible i.e. unadulterated, non-manufactured, and pure. Learn to become discerning with your food as much as possible, educating not only your sense of taste and smell, but your instinct. Note how each meal makes you feel and become more attuned to finding a balance with your foods. Try to avoid the tidal wave of manufactured dogma around foods and health because sadly, many people and even some doctors become caught up in the loop of misinformation and deception. Everything you place in your mouth is *your* responsibility and no one else's, as long as you are compos mentis. I suggest you go to the trouble of finding out which foods work best for you, (the metabolic typing model can be useful) and which to avoid. Being more discerning in the long term (at least 80-90% of the time) will help re-calibrate your instinct so you can reach the stage where you look at a food and know how it will make you feel, therefore assisting you to make better, or at least conscious, choices. That is where we all should naturally be.

Massage – ranges from the lightest skin stroking to skilled, remedial massage. When massage is given with wisdom, precision and skill, it goes a long way to ease tight muscles and re-balance soft tissues. Massage also contributes to relieving stress and re-balancing the autonomic nervous system. Not all massage treatments are equal and, even in these times of regulation; there is no guarantee of receiving an effective treatment. Only your instinct can tell you what will work best for you and who to go to.

Meditation – is often seen as a practice that must be worked at to bring the meditator back to a natural state of inner stillness or peace. Whilst this may be true to some degree, the effort implied could simply be ascribed to the ability to ignore the persistent thoughts that tend to bombard the human mind throughout his or her waking hours. The practice of meditation can be either active, as in the walking variety, or passive, and is often pursued in order to calm the autonomic nervous system and ease stress. However, Autogenics (see above) can be a good alternative to meditation. It is thought that caffeine inhibits the body's ability to achieve a theta (brainwave) state so may interfere with the ability to meditative.

Mercury toxicity – Mercury interferes with cellular activity and can be lodged in organs or tissues, impairing their normal function for years. Eating foods that boost your metabolism, removing blocking factors *and* detoxing your body can help free mercury and other toxins from the organs into the tissues for release from the body, but the process may be best done with the guidance of a nutritionist.

Metabolic Typing – a tailored eating plan, devised to re-balance your Autonomic Nervous System and maintain good health according to your genetic inheritance. An on-line test is used to determine your current autonomic status and makes recommendations based upon this aimed at strengthening your health. In time, and with practice, the concepts of this eating model can help to educate your natural ability to choose foods that make you feel well and stay well in the long term.

Milk – at its best when taken raw from pasture fed animals. Currently available from Hook & Sons via mail order (and a few others in the UK) as well as some farmers markets. See also www.chucklinggoat.co.uk.

Moderation – in everything helps achieve balance more easily. Imagine standing alone on the middle of a see-saw; placing a random weight on one end makes you work hard to balance; placing something measured on each end means little energy expenditure to retain balance. It's just the same within the body.

N

Natural – as in nature. Nature provides us with complete foods that we than put together. Manufacturers amalgamate unnatural elements to resemble food so we don't have to think. Choose wisely.

Nutritional information – checkout the **Weston A Price Foundation** for ongoing activities – see http://www.meetup.com/westonaprice-london/and the main WAPF website http://www.westonaprice.org/ for the low down on a healthy, mixed diet. WAPF have produced DVD sets of their London conferences with many eminent speakers talking about facts and misconceptions surrounding the food industry today. These are well worth getting if you want to take food choices and wisdom back into your own hands, especially if you have young children.

O

Organic food – check out the web for your local area. There's Abel & Cole and Riverford in the UK to name just a few, but local farming communities have other schemes too. Good Farmers' Markets exist in many areas now so support local produce where you can. It's a common fallacy that it's more expensive to eat only organic food; as it's naturally more nutrient dense, the body tends to be satisfied with less and does not continue to have cravings afterwards (because it's needs are met).

Overweight – The human body can only hold enough fuel for half a day - anything consumed over and above that amount will be accumulated as fat. If your system is in overload, it could be worth eating small meals for a while i.e. enough to sustain you, but less than a full meal, to allow your body to catch up on processing. Experimenting with macronutrient amounts (protein, fat, and carbohydrate) helps and has a direct effect upon your processing speed, commonly known as metabolism. If you want to know more about how foods affect our autonomic nervous system and metabolic rate, try exploring the metabolic typing model.

P

Parasites – are frequently overlooked as a cause of health problems and yet are extremely common amongst all cultures. They not only rob your body of vital nutrients, cause hormonal imbalances and sugar cravings, but their 'output' can cause serious toxic effects within your body as you play host to them. Gut ailments and sensitivities can be the result of parasites. Parasites are many and varied but the thing to remember is that they are expert at surviving and are therefore transmitted in ways that all of us can come into contact with. Following some sort of parasitic cleanse at least once a year is advisable for everyone. Allopathic or herbal formulations can be bought 'over the counter' in any chemist or health food shop. The most effective herbs are wormwood, black walnut and ground cloves. Seek the advice of a practitioner if in doubt.

Patience – an attribute that we all need to cultivate in order to reduce stress and develop a realistic perspective upon life. This takes mindfulness and a maturing attitude to life but brings an objectivity that cultivates wisdom over time.

Protein – is one of the three macronutrient groups that should form the basis of the human diet to provide the building blocks that our bodies need to maintain the cells, regulate its function and perform various metabolic functions every day. Even in civilized society, there are still many people who are confused by what protein is gained from, so may find themselves deficient without realizing it. The main symptoms of deficiency show as loss of muscle mass, fatigue, lethargy, irritability, apathy and protruding belly, not to mention severe dental caries. Protein deficiency in children means they fail to thrive or meet various developmental benchmarks such as reaching full size.

A lack of protein may also be a factor in poor sleeping ability as the body gets used to burning carbohydrates (which are used up quickly) and therefore wakes frequently seeking nourishment. An undernourished body cannot settle well.

A good visual cue to recognise lack of usable protein by the body is the quality of the hair; when it's very fine and seemingly weightless and dull, it would suggest there is insufficient keratin available (protein) to build a healthy hair shaft.

Q

Quality – make the quality of your food the best that you possibly can, assuming good health is your highest priority. After all, if the vessel (body) that carries your spirit is to provide you with the means to fulfil your choices, it needs to be in tip top condition. Whether you are a carnivore or vegetarian, make your protein and fat sources high quality and check out the best sources in your locality (although much can be obtained by post these days, including raw milk).

R

Raw foods – a gift from nature. Make good use of this highly prized resource to ensure you benefit from the complete nutrients available, before they are damaged or destroyed by heating. 40-50% raw is a good target to aim for.

Rebounder – is a small, firm trampoline; a wonderful aid to stimulating the lymphatic system and the corners of the mouth (turning them up), and a great way to exercise to your favourite music.

Reflux – a common condition whereby the contents of the stomach leak into the oesophagus, causing a burning pain. Interestingly, this can be a symptom of an autonomic nervous system imbalance which can be addressed by adjusting the diet. In general, it is not a case of the stomach being too acidic but rather the opposite, so antacids can make the problem worse. Lesser known is that this condition may also be improved by skilled abdominal massage that stretches and releases the fascia that's tight or snagging. See more in **digestion** above.

S

Senses – are how we experience the world around us. Dulling them with refined foods, chemical based products or lack of sleep can give us a very tepid view of life. When the senses are working as they designed to do, life is definitely more colourful.

Skin – the largest excretory organ of the body so needs to be toned like any other organs if it's to function well. A daily friction rub with a flannel whilst in the bath or shower stimulates the deeper levels of skin and also the lymphatic system; in my opinion, this is more effective than dry skin brushing.

Plastering products onto your skin that prevent sweating is much like wearing cling film; it might seem like a good idea at the time, but it causes more problems in the long run.

Sleep – is essential for good health, although for some needs to be worked at. I hope these suggestions help:

-

- It is best to go to bed being neither hungry nor full. You can't sleep restfully when you're hungry and get too hot from the energy produced by being full.

- Sleep cycles are 90 minutes long so setting your alarm to get you up in the middle of a cycle will have you feeling tired all day. For best results, get up at the end of a 90-minute cycle (i.e. after 6, 7.5 or even 9 hrs sleep).

- If you have difficulty getting to sleep because your head is full of thoughts, or if you frequently wake in the night and can't get back to sleep for the same reason, keep a note pad and pen by the bed to empty out the head, then sleep becomes easier. Your mind will keep you awake if it's holding on to stuff it thinks you need remember.

• Stay still if you can't get to sleep; every time you move, a dialogue between body and mind is renewed and the brain stays active. Not moving indicates to your mind that it's time to switch off.

• Go to bed before you're fit to drop. Avoid using up all the energy 'in the bank' and save some for the running repairs that need to happen while you sleep.

• Remember – a lack of sleep may not kill you, but the chemicals produced by stressing out over it just might. Relax and condition the mind to accept its situation. You might just be surprised by the result.

Stress – a little can be a good thing, but too much has been shown to consistently undermine health creating mild to severe problems. Stress is caused by two things; whether you *think* the unexpected situations around you cause fear/anxiety, then *how your body responds* to those thoughts. This mechanism is usually known as the 'fight or flight' response. Fight or flight triggers the release of key hormones – adrenalin and cortisol - that aid our survival, like being able to run faster or fight harder. Whilst various physiological changes occur to enable us to survive what was once a predatory lifestyle, the perceived threats are no longer of the advancing bear type and the response nowadays is triggered by more day-to-day events such as demanding children, traffic jams, a difficult boss or divorce.

Something else that is a factor in creating stress is not having the personal resources ie. the time or energy to manage your commitments.

The more often we experience the things we perceive as stressful, the more our stress levels are ramped up. Without regular exercise to burn off the extra hormones that our body produces for fight or flight, we begin to view the world as a hostile place, and spend a great deal of time either being defensive or overly sensitive and aggressive. So the stress level builds up, and the hormones continue to be produced, exhausting the adrenal glands. The long-term effect is to leave us being excitable, anxious, jumpy and irritable. This reduces our ability to work effectively. Focusing on survival means we make decisions based on the good of the self rather than the good of the group. We shut out information from other sources and cannot make balanced decisions.

Just as the causes are numerous, so are the solutions. As clarity is usually lacking when stress has accumulated, it can be helpful to seek the help of another to talk through your options, but in very simple terms, the following can be helpful:

- Check you are eating a balanced whole food diet at regular times
- Build a routine back into your life so you're not just being reactive
- Get enough sleep
- Take regular exercise to use up the extra cortisol in your body
- Learn a form of relaxation or meditation to calm your autonomic nervous system
- Do only what is necessary until you feel you're back on track.

Whilst it may at first seem arduous to orchestrate the above as you're having to be conscious of the changes you make, it will only be for a relatively short time. During this time, you'll be able to assess whether you're still aiming for the same goal in life or if you need to change it. Essentially, if you simplify your life until your energy has returned, you'll feel much clearer about what you want to keep in your life and what needs to go. When dealing with less of what you don't want and more of what you do want, your energy is far more likely to flow and life will take on a rosy glow.

Sunscreen – something that man devised so we could stay in the sun for unnaturally long periods, against our own better judgment or instinct. Many people have had the fear of God put into them about the effects of the sun, and wrongly so, probably because of manipulated or incorrect research. If we get back to common sense and realise that unless we are trekking across a desert, we can choose to limit the time we spend in the sun, build up our exposure gradually (yes, even in England, between the hours of 11am and 2pm, even when it's cloudy), and allow the skin to protect us naturally. Spending some time in the sun makes us feel better, uses up cholesterol and produces our much-needed Vitamin D. Many people now lack vitamin D and there are reports that rickets is re-emerging. Humans are meant to be free-range, not indoor reared, so exposing some skin to the sun/sky for around half an hour each day is indeed desirable.

Swimming – whilst being a fabulous form of exercise, unless done in fresh or sea water, it carries the problem of chlorine absorption. However, Dr Andrew Rostenburg (USA) claims that taking 500mg of Taurine before and after your dip can negate this problem.

T
Teeth – if you avoid eating fruit because of the effect the acid has on the enamel of your teeth, simply dissolve some bicarbonate of soda in a little water and swill out the mouth thoroughly to neutralize the acidic effect *after* eating the fruit. You could also try brushing your teeth with a little coconoil - this makes your teeth feel amazing.

Temperature – or thermoregulation. Why do some people feel the cold more than others? Whilst we may feel cold due to a shortage of Iodine in the body, the foods we eat can make a difference to how much heat we generate. Eating enough protein to build muscle helps because muscle generates heat. Also, how the Autonomic Nervous System is operating is important; being a para-sympathetic dominant diminishes the activity of the thyroid and therefore lowers the metabolic rate, whilst a heightened sympathetic response means improved thyroid function thus more heat being produced.

Therapies – there are lots of them, too numerous to mention. You do not have to place your faith in any one person or treatment and you may want to use several for different purposes at different times, but you must trust your instinct to tell you who and what is right for you. You will have a resonance with whoever you choose to work with that you will not find with everyone. Search until you feel 100% comfortable with your chosen therapist. Just be true to yourself and be happy with whatever you choose.

Thyroid function – lots of reading available on www.thyroiduk.org.uk. Some foods to avoid contain goitrogens (which slow down thyroid function) i.e. spinach and the brassica family (including the much heralded broccoli). Careful use of Lugol's Iodine improves thyroid function. See www.health-science-spirit.com

Time – is a precious thing. Take time to practice living in the now, rather than mentally racing ahead to the next distraction; that way, you will experience life more fully and perhaps make different choices because of this. Learn to meditate, to stretch your sense of time and become more present in each moment.

Traits – get to know your own. List your own strengths and weaknesses and think about how they can be used in order to take you towards your life goals. Of course they will change as you develop, or you may choose to change them.

Trying – can be used on a regular basis to balance the scales of self-esteem. If over-used, it can become a habit, a distraction and a stressor that uses up extraordinary amounts of energy. As most people wish to move towards their goals in life, a slightly different approach might be warranted, as in that of *choosing* what efforts to make in which direction, on a daily basis. Choosing is an option without an agenda, whereas it could be said that *trying* is to anticipate the outcome, with its accompanying expectations.

U
Undertow – be aware of consensus beliefs and try not to be dragged down by them. It can feel lonely to

have your own belief system but in time, this brings a strength of thinking, especially when you are confident that it is *your* truth. Undertow is most commonly but not exclusively felt through the media, so be discerning about what you choose to absorb or accept.

V

Variety – most definitely the spice of life! We find comfort in repeating the same choices on a regular basis, but having variety helps us be more conscious about the places we place ourselves in, and the choices we make in life.

Vegetarianism – is a choice that should be carefully thought out. Many teenagers take up the call as a stand for independence, without considering whether they are getting all the nutrients they need. Simply avoiding meat and filling the gap with 'anything' is not the answer. Some people do well as vegetarians, but not everyone. Humans are natural omnivores who require a mixed diet – at least some of which should be raw. Sadly, the last 20 years has seen a lack of education about what constitutes 'proper' food and the hype propagated by food conglomerates has become gospel. Nature knows how to produce food that contains all the nutrients we need – more of us need to remember how to use it properly again.

Vitamins – if you eat good quality fresh foods and your absorption is good, your need for supplements should be minimal. However for various reasons some may need supplements at certain times of their lives, and if so should ensure they are of good quality in order to do the job, for not all vitamins are equal.

W

Water – not only essential for life but necessary for effective digestion, and is a valuable conductor for conveying messages throughout the body.

Weight loss

We can lose excess body fat by using this suggested model that you control:

1. Write down 3 breakfasts – one light (fruit and natural yogurt), one starch based (i.e. porridge), and one protein based (less starch), whereby your choice is based upon:

   a) how you feel on that day and

   b) what your energetic expenditure is likely to be; more protein = more energy.

   Incorporate 1-2 tsp of coconoil for satiety and to crank up your metabolism. Remember, anything you do to increase your metabolic rate will help you to lose weight.

2. Spread your meals 3.5 - 4 hours apart, but no longer (unless you've been really sedentary and haven't finished digesting the previous meal). By doing this, you'll re-fuel before your blood sugar has dropped, thereby not feeling the need to eat as much and causing the body less stress. Remember, some people don't feel

hungry until they're ravenous, by which time you want to eat masses!

3. Don't eat beyond 1900 and get to bed before 2300.

Within – that curious place where the answers to anything we wish to know about ourselves can be found.

Y

Yoga – a wonderful practice for stretching, tuning and balancing the physical form. Because of the emphasis on breathing, it also acts as a sort of moving meditation, bringing symbiosis to mind and body. Yoga stimulates the autonomic nervous system, hence it's balancing effect.

Further reading

Louise L. Hay, *You can Heal your Body*

Candace B. Pert, *Molecules of Emotion*

Bruce H. Lipton, *The Biology of Belief*

Donna Eden, *Energy Medicine for Women*

Donna Eden, *The Little Book of Energy Medicine*

Lauren Walker, *Energy Medicine Yoga*

James L. Oschman, *Energy Medicine – The Scientific Basis*

Jean-Pierre Barral, *Understanding the Messages of Your Body*

Margaret McCarthy, *Lymphatic Therapy for Toxic Decongestion*

Henry Lindlahr, *Philosophy of Natural Therapeutics*

Shawn Talbott, *The Cortisol Connection*

Doc Childre & Howard Martin, *The HeartMath Solution*

W. Walcott & Trish Fahey, *The Metabolic Typing Diet*

Sally Fallon, *Nourishing Traditions*

Brigitte Mars, *Rawsome*

Shawn Talbott, *The Cortisol Connection*

Henry G. Bieler, *Food is Your Best Medicine*

Gary Taubes, *The Diet Delusion*

Lynda Bunnell & Ra Uru Hu, *The Definitive Book of Human Design*

Robert Fritz, The *Path of Least Resistance*

Tom Campbell, *My Big Toe.*

Thinking of You

When form doth feel and heart doth ache,
When aches and pains each moment make,
When heaviness doth overtake
The energy of You.

When mind forgets its purpose here,
Digestion falters and appear
More problems than you'd care to hear –
Then think again of You.

Recall the time when in your youth
Your energy was not your truth,
For youth is oft beyond reproof –
So think now of You.

The care for soul and vessel takes
More time than we're prepared to make,
But trust in this for your own sake
If you value You.

Each moment that you put back in
To balance all that's in your skin
Will fill your heart as you begin
The tender care of You.

Let balance be your only goal,
So meditate and fill your soul
Until you feel like you are whole
In memory of You.

AGD 2012

About the Author

Angela was born with a natural curiosity that has led her to explore many subjects, leading to a diverse knowledge on matters of health. She is quick to see the potential in the individuals she meets and is keen to shine a light on their path, showing what is possible should they wish to explore that direction.

Whilst Angela's life has presented situations that have merited a great deal of exploration, her approach has always been to gain the wider picture then to distil the ensuing knowledge and experience down to small practical nuggets that anyone can try for him or herself. Being a very practical person, Angela's delivery always aims to be concise, accessible and adaptable but without spoon-feeding *all* the answers, because as individuals we each have our own unique solutions.

As a skilled massage therapist of some 25 years, it is common during treatment for Angela to share her knowledge and experience, always aiming to help clients to better long term health and a happier life. The repeated requests to write this information down brought this book into being, for as humans, it is so easy to forget the little things that can make our lives easier.

Now, in an age where people are more educated in self-care, whilst bodywork is still required, Angela's work has shifted to include coaching and Soul Plan reading in order to help people visualise their own big picture and where they are in it, opening the door to the many choices that lead to their own potential.

147